Clinical Nursing Manual

Edited by Jennifer E. Clark

Deputy Director of Nurse Education, Queen
Elizabeth School of Nursing, Birmingham

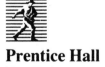

Prentice Hall

New York   London   Toronto   Sydney   Tokyo   Singapore

First published 1990 by
Prentice Hall International (UK) Ltd,

66 Wood Lane End, Hemel Hempstead,
Hertfordshire, HP2 4RG
A division of
Simon & Schuster International Group

Printed and bound in Great Britain
by Dotesios Printers Ltd, Trowbridge, Wiltshire.

British Library Cataloguing in Publication Data

Clark, Jennifer E.
  Clinical nursing manual.
  1. Medicine, Nursing
  I. Title
  610.73

  ISBN 0–13–137811–2

1 2 3 4 5 94 93 92 91 90

*To past, present and future patients of
Central Birmingham Health Authority
without whom there would be no purpose
to this book.*

Contents

Foreword

Practising nurses everywhere, both in community and hospital settings, are trying to give the best possible care to their clients and patients within an environment which, more than ever before, seems to be governed by limited resources and an ever-growing demand for service. Increasing dependency levels, shorter hospital stay and earlier discharge into the community are the norm, influencing each aspect of the nurse's role, as practitioner, educator or manager.

In addition, each nurse is charged with ensuring that their practice reflects up-to-date knowledge and relevant research findings, not an easy task in today's nursing world.

This book has been produced as a joint venture by nurses working within clinical areas of Central Birmingham Health Authority and Queen Elizabeth School of Nursing. They are well used to the realities of today's NHS and have combined forces to provide a valuable source of information for colleagues who, like them, strive to provide the best care under demanding circumstances and who need to have access to research-based nursing practices which also reflect a process approach to care.

I am personally indebted to them for the many hours of work they have contributed in order to enhance patient and client care and can commend this book, the outcome of their efforts, to you.

Mrs Lyn Copcutt (B. Ed. (Hons), Postgraduate
Certificate in Education, Diploma in Nursing,
Postgraduate Diploma in Psychology, RGN)

Director of Nurse Education
Queen Elizabeth School of Nursing
Birmingham

Membership of Central Birmingham Nursing Procedure Committee

Chairperson: Jennifer Clark. M.Sc. Certificate in Education, SRN, SCM, HV.Cert., RNT, Deputy Director of Nurse Education, Queen Elizabeth School of Nursing.

Secretary: Maggie Reeves, RGN, RM, Dip.N. (London), Certificate in Education, RCNT, Clinical Teacher, Queen Elizabeth School of Nursing.

Patricia Stevens, B.Ed.(Hons), Certificate in Education. Dip.N.(London), RNT, RGN, ND N.Cert., Nurse Tutor, Queen Elizabeth School of Nursing.

Donna Winning, RGN, ND N.Cert., RCNT, Nursing Developments Officer, Queen Elizabeth Hospital.

Jean Mandefield, RGN, DNC OND, Nursing Officer, Central Birmingham Health Authority, Community.

Jo Manion, SRN, RCNT, Diploma in Orthopaedic Nursing, Clinical Teacher, Queen Elizabeth School of Nursing.

Christabel Norman, SRN, RCNT, Clinical Teacher, Queen Elizabeth School of Nursing.

Lynette Hollick, RMN, DPSN, Nursing Officer, Mental Health Unit, Central Birmingham Health Authority.

Pamela Done, SRN, SCM, Ward Sister, The Women's Hospital, Birmingham.

Judith Wedgwood, RGN, Certificate in Education, DPSN ENB Course 100, Clinical Nurse Specialist in Nutrition, Queen Elizabeth Hospital.

Lesley Callinan, SRN, RSCN, Ward Sister, The General Hospital, Birmingham.

Pauline Hobbs, SRN, OHN Cert., District Clinical Nurse Specialist, Infection Control.

Preface

This book has arisen as a result of one Health Authority's dissatisfaction with its clinical nursing procedures. The introduction of the nursing process, nursing models and primary nursing, all of which stress the individuality of the patient, led to an outcry of discontent towards the existing nursing procedures which were prescriptive in style and left very little opportunity for flexibility of approach.

In 1987, a new procedure committee was formed within Central Birmingham Health Authority whose remit it was to rewrite all the nursing procedures under a new format. It was determined that this format would achieve the following objectives:

1. Provide broad principles or guidelines for care rather than prescriptive detail, which would allow greater flexibility for the nurse.
2. Reflect the stages of the nursing process and thus an individualised approach to care.
3. Provide a rationale for all the principles given, which would assist nurses, especially learner nurses, to fully understand the care they give.

As a committee we felt it essential to build our new procedures on current research findings. A computerised and manual literature search was conducted for each procedure. Where relevant research has been found this has been incorporated into practice and referenced at the conclusion of each chapter.

The Health Authority is designated as a teaching authority which provides a wide range of both specialist and general nursing care. Most of the procedures described in the narrative would be of relevance to any health authority wishing to adopt a more flexible research-based approach to their nursing practice.

It has been the aim throughout to improve the nursing care given to patients, whilst still ensuring accuracy and safety for the patient and nurse. At times this has proved to be a difficult task; however, comments from the clinical staff towards the new procedures have been very positive.

The nature of nursing requires its practitioners to constantly reflect, review and revise their practice to ensure that the best possible standard of care is given to patients. We believe that the principles of care outlined within this manual make an excellent foundation for practice, but as Winston Churchill said

> This is not the end. It is not even the beginning of the end. But it is, perhaps, the end of the beginning. (1942)

Acknowledgements

The Procedure Committee of Central Birmingham Health Authority would like to express our thanks to the Queen Elizabeth School of Nursing secretarial staff with special thanks to Mrs Pamela Techene for so painstakingly typing the manuscript. This has necessitated many hours spent at the word processor, both in typing the first draft and then re-editing and we have all been impressed by her patience and willingness to see the project through to a successful conclusion.

Our thanks go also to Mr Stephen Gough (Librarian) and Mrs Shirley Harris (Library Assistant) for checking so many of the references provided throughout the narrative.

We would also like to thank the following members of nursing staff who have individually contributed specific procedures: Mrs Margaret Berker, Nurse Teacher, QESN; Mrs Elaine Cook, Nurse Teacher, QESN; Mrs Carol Dealey, Clinical Teacher and Clinical Nurse Specialist in Tissue Viability, CBHA; Miss Kathy Lowe, Nurse Teacher, QESN; Mrs Wendy Pringle, Clinical Nurse Specialist in Stoma Care, CBHA.

Our thanks go also to the staff of CBHA Supplies Department and to the staff of the Queen Elizabeth Hospital Pharmacy and Physiotherapy Departments for their advice and help with specific procedures.

Finally, we acknowledge that there are many other teaching and nursing colleagues too numerous to mention who have helped and encouraged us by giving their expertise and support. To them we extend a very special note of gratitude.

List of figures and tables

Figures

Tables

Specific principles underlying all the procedures

The following principles should be applied to each of the procedures contained within the manual:

1. Nurses should wash hands thoroughly before and after each procedure. The use of an alcohol hand rub may substitute hand washing when hands become inadvertently contaminated during a procedure.

2. Patients should be offered handwashing facilities where appropriate and especially after using the toilet, commode or bedpan.

3. Nurses' uniforms should be protected with a plastic disposable apron when performing procedures and they must be changed between dirty and clean procedures.

4. All equipment used for patient care should be maintained in a hygienic condition and cleaned between patient use. Please refer to Health Authority disinfection policy.

5. All waste and used linen should be disposed of with minimal handling in designated containers. Please refer to Health Authority waste/linen policy.

6. To ensure patient and staff safety, nursing equipment should not be placed or left on the floor.

7. To ensure patient safety, nursing staff should adhere to the Health Authority uniform policy with special reference to the wearing of jewellery and the care of finger-nails.

8. All the procedures contained within the book can cause pain or discomfort, loss of dignity or embarrassment. Therefore, a well-informed consent should be obtained wherever possible from the patient prior to commencement of the procedure.

1   Abdominal paracentesis

Definition

Insertion of a small trochar or cannula through the abdominal wall into the peritoneal cavity for diagnostic or therapeutic reasons.

Assessment

Action	Rationale
Determine reason for procedure:	To ensure appropriate preparation of patient and equipment.
• To remove ascitic fluid in order to relieve pressure which interferes with respiration or bladder function. • To obtain a specimen for cytological examination. • To introduce drugs.	
Assess condition of patient.	To facilitate correct positioning of patient without causing further discomfort. To facilitate adequate explanation of procedure and reduction of anxiety.

Planning

Equipment

Trolley.
Sterile abdominal paracentesis set containing: trochar and cannula, rubber tubing, scalpel and surgical blade, gallipot and cotton wool.

5 ml syringe and needles.
Local anaesthetic.
Antiseptic solution.
Sterile gloves.
Safety pins.
Sterile drainage bag and holder.
Gate clip/clamp.
Waterproof plaster.
Disposal bag.
Sterile specimen pots and laboratory forms.

Action	Rationale
Explain the procedure to the patient.	To obtain the co-operation and consent of patient.
Ask patient to empty bladder.	Risk of bladder being punctured by cannula if it is full.
Measure patient's girth.	To have comparable measurements before and after procedure – to facilitate assessment of fluid loss.
Place patient in a comfortable position – usually sitting up or semi-recumbent.	This position will facilitate drainage of fluid.
Rearrange bedclothes.	To maintain patient's dignity.
Cleanse and prepare trolley.	To prevent infection.

Implementation

Action	Rationale
Reassure and observe patient during procedure.	To reduce anxiety and maintain patient co-operation throughout the procedure.

To monitor patient's condition. |
| Assist doctor as required with obtaining specimens. | To aid early diagnosis. |
| Apply gate clip to tubing of drainage system. | To control flow of ascitic fluid. Flow must be reduced after 1 litre has drained as there is a risk of shock. |

Reposition patient on to side of cannula when flow is diminishing.	To facilitate drainage of fluid.
Ensure that a dry dressing which is secure and supports the cannula is *in situ*.	To protect wound site from contamination. Prevent dislodging of cannula.
Support tubing.	To prevent dislodging of cannula when patient moves.
Measure girth.	To enable medical staff to compare previous measurement and assess fluid loss.

Evaluation

Potential problems of procedure	Appropriate nursing action
Shock. Sudden change in intra-abdominal pressure may cause vasodilation and a fall in blood pressure.	Stop flow of ascitic fluid by clamping off drainage tube with gate clip/clamp. Record vital signs. Report at once to medical staff.
Dehydration and electrolyte imbalance.	Monitor fluid balance. Encourage oral fluids.
Lowered plasma proteins.	Encourage a high protein diet.
Cessation of drainage.	Change position of patient. 'Milking' tubing may remove possible clots. Change drainage system. Inform medical staff.
Infection.	Observe temperature whilst cannula is *in situ*. Observe cannula site. Obtain swab for culture. Report to medical staff.

Adaptations for home care

This is a medical procedure and will only be undertaken in the community in order to relieve pressure.

Planning

1. Agree time and date for procedure with general practitioner, patient and carer.
2. Arrange delivery of abdominal paracentesis set from Central Sterile Supply Department (CSSD).
3. Obtain prescription for local anaesthetic from general practitioner.
4. Remaining equipment should be taken from the clinic to the patient's home by the district nurse.
5. Prepare and protect agreed working surface.
6. On completion of procedure, carer should be advised to contact the general practitioner immediately if they are worried about the patient's condition.
7. Return all used equipment from pack to CSSD immediately after use.

References and further reading

Phipps, W.J. (1980), *Shafer's Medical–Surgical Nursing*, 7th edn, p. 550.

2 Admission to hospital

Definition

Planned admission

An admission that has been pre-arranged and prepared for by the hospital and patient. It usually ensures that the patient has personal effects and friends and relatives are aware.

Emergency admission

An admission brought about by accident or sudden onset of illness. Relatives are often unaware and the patient may be without personal effects.

Aim

The aim of the nurse should be to lessen the negative effects of admission by clear, concise, empathetic verbal and non-verbal communication with both the patient and their relatives, taking into consideration age, gender and cultural background.

Assessment

Action	Rationale
Follow admission procedure for your ward/department.	To ensure continuity.
Assess mental and physical condition of patient.	To ensure that the patient is not put in the 'sick role' unnecessarily.
Assess patient's understanding of reason for admission.	To alleviate fear and anxiety.

Assess the patient's ability to provide information.

To ensure that the patient does not become distressed or over-exerted.

To ensure that accurate information is provided.

Determine the presence of friends or relatives.

The accompanying person may give support and/or provide information the nurse requires.

Determine the reason for admission and any instructions from the admitting medical officers.

To ensure that the patient receives the correct treatment.

Assess order of priorities.

To facilitate discharge planning.
met.

Be aware of nursing assessment detail and factors which could affect discharge.

To avoid needless questioning.

To facilitate discharge planning.

Planning

Assemble equipment.

To ensure safe accurate and comfortable nursing care is given.

Obtain the medical record folder.

To gain factual details, thus avoiding repetitious questions.

To determine diagnosis and any medical instructions which may not have been given verbally.

Assemble nursing record documents.

To facilitate individualised patient care and to meet UKCC requirements.

Ensure name and number band is in place and matches medical record folder.

For correct identification of patient.

Implementation

Identify and greet patient introducing yourself.

First impressions can affect a patient's or relative's opinion.

Assume a friendly approach to patients and relatives.	To ensure that they feel welcome.
Avoid use of abbreviations or jargon.	Can confuse and belittle a patient.
Allow opportunities for questions.	To decrease anxiety.
Accompany patient and companion to bed space.	The bed space becomes the patient's 'home'. It is important that they are only moved when this is essential.
Assist patient to get undressed and into bed if necessary.	To give patient maximum comfort. It is difficult to accept the 'sick role' when well and needing minor surgery.
Check that companion and patient are aware of essential information, e.g. visiting times, ward name and phone number.	To reduce anxiety levels.
Ensure all property and valuables are checked, documented and stored according to Health Authority policy.	To assure safety and minimise risk of theft.
Determine if patient is taking any medication. Record details on nursing records.	May facilitate continuity or review of treatment.
Store medication according to Health Authority policy.	To ensure correct storage or disposal.
Ensure *relevant* personal details are recorded in nursing records, e.g. next of kin.	To ensure speedy communication of essential information.
Ensure appropriate orientation to ward is given, e.g. explain the call bell/light systems.	Anxiety or pain reduces ability to retain information. To minimise the sense of isolation.
Explain ward personnel and introduce neighbouring patients.	To reduce confusion and emphasise sense of belonging.
Explain relevant ward layout and policies.	To help reduce misunderstanding and also maintain safety.

Complete nursing documentation at the earliest opportunity, avoiding a stereotyped approach.

To provide a written baseline of the individual patient's condition on admission.

To facilitate free flow of relevant information.

Carry out relevant observations, explaining their necessity.

To provide accurate baseline data and to detect any actual or potential abnormalities.

To reduce anxiety levels.

Evaluation

Potential problems of procedure

Patient's anxiety.

Appropriate nursing action

Give support and information to reduce anxiety.

Involve support personnel as appropriate.

Monitor degree of anxiety.

Adaptation for home care

This procedure is not relevant in the community.

References and further reading

Lelliot, P. (1986), 'First impressions', *The Health Service Journal*, June, p. 829.

Nolan, N. (1986), 'Can someone please explain it all to me?' *Health & Social Service Journal*, 2 January, p. 16.

Pearson, M. (1986), 'Fitting in', *Senior Nurse*, vol. 4(6), pp. 14–15.

Price, R. (1983), 'Just a few forms to fill in', *Nursing Times*, vol. 79(44), pp. 26–8. Particularly refer to cartoon.

Shillitoe, R. (1985), 'I think, therefore I'm ill', *Nursing Times*, vol. 81(8), pp. 24–6.

Smeltzer, C.H. and Flores, S.M. (1986), 'Pre-admission discharge planning', *Journal of Nursing Administration*, vol. 16(5), pp. 14–15.

Wilson-Barnett, J. (1976), 'Patients' emotional reactions to hospitalisation: an exploratory study', *Journal of Advanced Nursing*, vol. 1(5), pp. 351–8.

Wilson-Barnett, J. (1978), 'In hospital: patients' feelings and opinions', *Nursing Times*, Occasional papers, vol. 74(8), pp. 29–32.

3   Apex beat/radial pulse recording

Definition

The simultaneous counting of the radial pulse and the left ventricle of the heart by two nurses.

Aim

To compare the apical contractions with the radial beats for any pulse deficit.

Assessment

Action	Rationale
Assess the condition of the patient.	To facilitate appropriate explanation of the procedure and to gain the patient's co-operation.
Ascertain the reason for and the frequency of the recordings.	To monitor the patient's condition without causing undue disturbance.

Planning

This procedure always requires two nurses.

Equipment

    Watch with a second hand.
    Stethoscope.
    Appropriate chart.
    Red and blue pens.

Action	**Rationale**
Screen bed and expose area of chest required for taking apex beat.	To ensure privacy and to be able to hear the apex beat.
Place the watch in a convenient position.	To enable both nurses to see the watch and to begin and end their counting at a predetermined time.

Implementation

Action	**Rationale**
Place diaphragm of stethoscope at the fifth intercostal space, 5 cm to the left of the sternum.	To facilitate hearing and counting of the ventricular contractions.
Second nurse palpates radial pulse.	To facilitate the procedure.
At a given time, both nurses begin counting for exactly 1 min.	By counting concurrently, differences in apical and radial rates can be detected.
Record both apical and radial pulses clearly, e.g. using different colours or symbols.	To differentiate between the two recordings.
Make patient comfortable and remove the screens from around the patient.	

Evaluation

Potential problems of procedure	**Appropriate Nursing action**
Difficulty in hearing apical beat.	Place diaphragm of stethoscope approximately between the sixth and seventh rib, 5–10 cm to the left of the sternum.
	N.B. In severe pulmonary oedema it may be impossible to hear the apical beat accurately.

Adaptations for home care

Procedure is conducted as outlined above.

References and Further Reading

Jamieson, E., McCall, J. and Blythe, R. (1988), *Guidelines for Clinical Nursing Practices*, Churchill Livingstone, Edinburgh, pp. 82–3.
Pritchard, A.P. and Walker, V.A. (eds.) (1984), *The Royal Marsden Hospital Manual of Clinical Nursing Policies and Procedures*, Harper & Row, London, pp. 353–4.

4   Barrier nursing (source isolation)

Definition

The means of isolating an infected patient who could be a risk to others.

Aim

To confine the organisms and block the route of spread. This procedure should be read in conjunction with the Prevention of Cross-Infection procedure in Chapter 16.

Assessment

Action	Rationale
Determine the source and route of infection.	To ensure the appropriate precautions are taken.

Planning

N.B. A single room is desirable.

Equipment

Trolley or table.
Unsterile disposable gloves and aprons.
Sharps container ⎫
Rubbish bags   ⎬ as required (see Table 16.1)
Linen bags   ⎭
Soap.
Alcohol hand rub.
Recording charts.
For basic nursing equipment see Table 16.1.

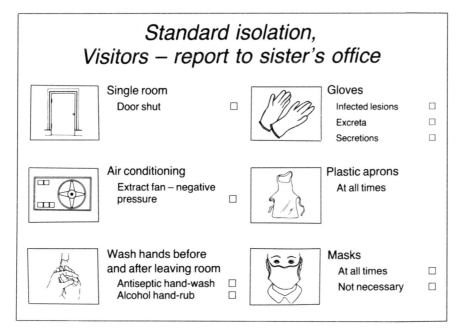

Figure 4.1 Standard isolation chart.

Notice stating that visitors must report to nurse in charge and listing precautions to be taken.

Action	Rationale
Place notice on outside of door.	To inform anyone entering the room about the type of barrier nursing that is in progress, ensuring that people do not enter the room unnecessarily.
Set up the trolley/table outside door with aprons, gloves, alcohol hand rub and recording charts.	To ensure that people entering room will have appropriate equipment available and that charts can be viewed without entering room.
Ensure that hand washing facilities are available.	To prevent the spread of organisms.
Place patient's property and equipment (e.g. washbowl), inside room.	Equipment used by patient will be contaminated.

Place appropriate rubbish/linen bags in room (see Table 16.1).	To prevent spread of organisms and ensure safety.
Place designated rigid container for sharp objects in room as required.	To prevent spread of organisms and ensure safety.
Explain procedure to patient and relatives.	To reduce anxiety and gain co-operation,

Implementation

Before entering room:

- Put on a plastic apron.
- Wash hands (or alcohol rub).
- Put on gloves if required.

To prevent contamination of clothing.

To prevent contamination of hands.

On entering the room shut the door.	To prevent spread of organisms and hazard to others.
Place used linen in appropriate bags according to Health Authority policy. Prior to collection, both the inner and outer protective bag should be securely tied. Label accordingly.	To prevent spread of organisms and hazard to others.
Place rubbish/soiled dressings in appropriate bag. The top of the bag should be tightly closed before leaving room.	To prevent spread of organisms and hazard to others.
Dispose of all rubbish and linen on a frequent basis.	To prevent buildup of rubbish and linen, which could be a source of infection within the patient's room.

Carefully dispose of excreta by:

To prevent spread of organisms through excreta.

- Covering bed pan.
- Removing immediately.
- Cleansing/destroying bedpan.
- Returning cleansed receptacle to room.

Remove apron and gloves before leaving room. Discard in appropriate bag.	To prevent the spread of organisms.
Wash hands.	To remove harmful organisms from hands.
Leave room, shutting door.	To contain organisms.
Rinse hands with alcohol rub.	To remove remaining organisms.
When patient is discharged, ensure the room is cleansed according to Health Authority policy.	To remove contaminants from surfaces.

Evaluation

Potential problems of procedure	**Appropriate nursing action**
Physical and social isolation for patient.	Provide patient with appropriate entertainment activities, e.g. television, reading material.
	Keep patient informed of rationale for procedure.
	Spend time listening and talking to patient whilst giving care.
	Encourage close relatives to visit and participate in care, having learnt barrier nursing technique.
Staff anxiety.	Ensure all staff are adequately informed of procedure.
Routine cleaning of room.	Ensure domestic staff are aware of precautions to take. For specific cases refer to infection control nursing officer.

Adaptation for home care

The principles of the above procedure could be applied in the community, e.g. when nursing a child with an infectious disease.

5 Reverse barrier nursing (protective isolation)

Definition

The means of protecting a susceptible patient from infection. This procedure should be read in conjunction with the Prevention of Cross-Infection procedure in Chapter 16.

Assessment

Action	Rationale
Identify patient at risk.	To ensure the appropriate precautions are taken.
Identify the reason for isolation.	To adapt the procedure to the specific needs of the patient's condition.

Planning

N.B. A single room is essential.

Equipment

Notice on door stating that all visitors/staff should report to nurse in charge (see Figure 5.1).
Plastic apron.
Soap and paper towels.
Alcohol hand rub.
Basic nursing equipment (see Table 16.1) should be patient-designated.

Action	Rationale
Ensure the room and equipment are cleansed thoroughly before use according to Health Authority policy.	To reduce the number of organisms present.

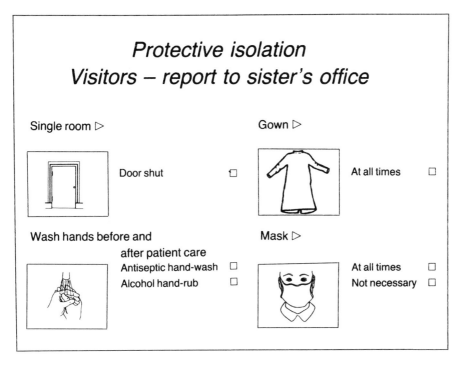

Figure 5.1 Protective isolation chart.

Explain procedure to patient and relatives.

Reduce anxiety and gain co-operation.

Limit the number of visitors according to ward policy and condition of patient.

Identified visitors minimise the risk of infection.

N.B. Visitors and staff should not attend patient if they have been in contact with an infectious disease to which they are susceptible or have an infection, e.g. herpes, septic lesions, diarrhoea and vomiting, etc.

Place notice on outside of door.

To inform anyone entering the room the type of barrier nursing which is in progress, ensuring that people do not enter the room unnecessarily.

Implementation

Wash hands thoroughly and put on apron before dealing with patient.	Organisms may be transferred from the hands or clothing.
Record temperature and pulse every 4 hours and check for any signs of infection.	To aid early detection of infection.

Evaluation

Potential problem of procedure	Appropriate nursing action
Physical and social isolation.	Provide patient with appropriate entertainment activities, e.g. television, reading material.
	Spend time listening and talking to the patient whilst giving care.
	Encourage previously identified visitors to participate in care.
	Keep patient informed of the rationale for procedure.

Adaptations for home care

The principles of the above procedure could be applied in the community.

References and further reading

Acquired Infection in the NHS and its Prevention, Royal College of Nursing, 1978.

Ayliffe, G.A.J., Collins, B.J. and Taylor, L.J. (1982), *Hospital Acquired Infection – Principles and Prevention*, Wright & Sons, Bristol.

Bagshawe, K.D. (1978), 'Isolating patients in hospital to control infection', *British Medical Journal*, vol. 2, pp. 609–12.

Central Birmingham District Control of Infection Policy.

Central Birmingham Health Authority Disinfectant and Antiseptic Policy.

Lowbury, E.J.L., Ayliffe, G.A.J., Geddes, A.M. and Williams, J.D. (1981), *Control of Hospital Infection*, 2nd edn, Chapman & Hall, London.

Maurer, I.M. (1985), *Hospital Hygiene*, 3rd edn, Edward Arnold, London.

6   Bathing

Definition

Bathing the patient in bathroom, shower or bed. A means of cleansing the patient in the appropriate location.

Aim

To promote a feeling of well-being, comfort and cleanliness.

Assessment

Action	Rationale
Determine the patient's preference regarding time and location of procedure.	To endorse the patient's feeling of independence.
Ascertain the amount of help required by the patient.	To maintain safety.
	To select appropriate equipment.
	To facilitate independence.

Planning

Equipment

Patient's toiletries (if necessary, supply from ward stores).
Appropriately sized towels.
Patient's own bowl (if washed beside or in bed).

Action	Rationale
Ensure privacy can be maintained and that the appropriate location is warm, clean and tidy. The floor should be dry at all times.	To maintain a safe environment and to promote comfort.
N.B. If patient is bathed in bed remove excess bedclothes, but ensure patient remains covered and warm. If patient has been incontinent, cleanse patient appropriately before commencement of procedure.	
Offer toilet facilities prior to procedure.	To maintain patient comfort and reduce anxiety.
Ensure temperature of water is acceptable to the patient (test with forearm), approximately 40°C.	To promote patient comfort.
N.B. When filling bath, add hot water to cold.	To maintain a safe environment.
Check the patient's needs for pain control.	Movement may cause further pain and reduce the patient's ability to co-operate.
Explain equipment (if used) to the patient.	To reduce anxiety, e.g. if ambulift is used.

Implementation

Action	Rationale
Ensure privacy is maintained throughout.	To promote patient dignity.
Assist patient to wash giving the appropriate amount of help as ascertained in assessment.	To maintain independence.
Check, adjust and apply brakes on all equipment for optimum safety and comfort throughout.	To avoid injury to staff and patient.

Ensure the patient is comfortable at all times.

Be as quick as possible when washing the patient, only exposing those areas being washed.

To prevent chilling the patient and to maintain dignity.

Listen and talk to the patient throughout procedure.

Patients often reveal problems to nurses when intimate tasks are being performed.

Observe patient's hair and nails and all areas of skin when washing.

To detect any abnormalities (see Pressure Area Care procedure in Chapter 42).

Change the water as often as possible.

To promote patient comfort.

After use, clean and dry all equipment and store according to Health Authority policy.

To prevent cross-infection.

Offer the patient facilities to clean their teeth, shave, comb hair and apply make-up.

To promote self-esteem.

When using an ambulift, the arms of the ambulift may be removed whilst patient is in the bath.

To enable patient to have movement whilst in the bath.

The arms of the ambulift should not be placed on the floor and should be replaced before removing patient from bath.

To prevent cross-infection and avoid accidents.

Evaluation

Potential problem of procedure

Hypothermia, especially in the elderly.

Appropriate nursing action

Check patient is warm on completion of the procedure.

If necessary provide extra heating/ bedclothes.

Adaptations for home care

The procedure is conducted as outlined above, ensuring an adequate supply of hot water, towels and clean clothes prior to commencement.

References and further reading

Ayliffe, G.A.J., Collins, B.J. and Taylor, L.J. (1982), *Hospital Acquired Infection – Principles and Prevention*, Wright & Sons, Bristol.
Dealey, C. and Berker, M. (1986), 'Action speaks louder than words', *Nursing Times*, vol. 82(29), pp. 37–9.
Greaves, A. (1985), 'We'll just freshen you up dear' *Nursing Times*, vol. 27(6), pp. 3–8.
Joynson, D.H.M. (1978), 'Bowls and bacteria', *Journal of Hygiene*, vol. 80(423), pp. 423–5.

7   Biopsy

Definition

To obtain a specimen of body tissue for microscopic examination. N.B. For specific aspects of each procedure refer to grid.

Assessment

Action	Rationale
Determine the physical and psychological condition of the patient.	To ensure that a comfortable, appropriate position is assumed and that information is given at a level that the patient understands.

Planning

Equipment

Trolley.
Sterile biopsy needle of appropriate type.
Dressing packs.
Dressing towel.
Sterile syringes 20, 10 and 2 ml.
Assorted needles.
One pair of sterile surgeon's gloves.
One occlusive dressing.
Alcohol-based cleansing lotion.
Local anaesthetic, e.g. lignocaine 1 per cent.
Disposal bag.
Laboratory form.
Appropriate specimen container/slides.

N.B. Refer to Tables 7.1 to 7.4 for specific equipment.

Table 7.1 Pleural biopsy

Assessment	Planning	Implementation	Evaluation
Record base line observations of temperature, pulse, respirations and blood pressure.	Specific equipment required: pleural biopsy needle.	Position patient upright, leaning forward over a bed table, supported by a pillow.	Close observation of respiration, blood pressure and pulse, due to the risk of a pneumothorax.

Table 7.2 Renal biopsy

Assessment	Planning	Implementation	Evaluation
Record base line observations of temperature, pulse and blood pressure. Assess the ability of the patient to lie prone.	Specific equipment required: renal biopsy needle.	Position the patient prone with one pillow. Assist in the application of a pressure dressing to wound following procedure. The patient is nursed on bedrest according to doctor's instructions, e.g. 24 hours.	Close observation of pulse, blood pressure, temperature, wound site, urinary output and haematuria due to risk of haemorrhage and/or seepage of urine.

Table 7.3 Bone marrow aspiration

Assessment	Planning	Implementation	Evaluation
Identify site to be used, e.g. sternum, iliac crest. Determine if sedation is to be given.	Specific equipment required: bone marrow aspiration needle, 4–6 glass slides, dry, protective sterile containers.	Position patient appropriately according to collection site. Sternum: supine with one pillow. Iliac crest: right or left lateral. Apply pressure to the site for approximately 15 min. Apply a dry dressing after 15 min if no bleeding apparent.	Close observation of temperature and pulse due to the risk of infection, and blood pressure due to the risk of haemorrhage.

Table 7.4 Liver biopsy

Assessment	Planning	Implementation	Evaluation
Record base line observation of blood pressure and pulse. Determine if sedation is to be given.	Specific equipment required: liver biopsy needle; sterile container and transport medium.	Place patient in supine position with one pillow. Their right side should be proximal to the edge of the bed. Instruct the patient to take a deep breath and hold it whilst the biopsy is being taken. The patient is nursed on bedrest according to doctor's instructions, e.g. for 6 hours.	Close observation of pulse, blood pressure and wound site, due to the high risk of haemorrhage.

Action	**Rationale**
Explain the procedure and the purpose of the procedure to the patient.	To gain consent and co-operation.

Implementation

N.B. This procedure is carried out by the medical staff, assisted by the nurse, whose main responsibility is to the patient at all times.

Action	**Rationale**
Prepare the trolley, dressing pack and supplementary items.	To facilitate the procedure.
Observe and comfort the patient throughout the procedure.	To reduce distress.
Assist the doctor as required throughout the procedure.	To facilitate a swift and easy procedure.
When the needle is withdrawn, assist in the application of an occlusive dressing.	To prevent micro-organisms entering the wound site.

Ensure that the specimen is deposited in/on the appropriately labelled container/slide.	To prevent degeneration of specimen and unnecessary repetition of the procedure.
Ensure the specimen is transported as quickly as possible to the appropriate laboratory.	To prevent degeneration of specimen and unnecessary repetition of the procedure.

For specific aspects of implementation refer to Tables 7.1 to 7.4.

Evaluation

Potential problem of procedure	Appropriate nursing action
Pain at biopsy site.	Give prescribed analgesia.
	Monitor effectiveness.
	Inform medical staff appropriately.

For specific problems refer to Tables 7.1 to 7.4.

Adaptations for home care

This procedure is not relevant to the community.

References and further reading

Watson, J. and Royle, J. (1987), *Watson's Medical and Surgical Nursing and Related Physiology*, 3rd edn, Bailliere Tindal, London.

8   Bladder irrigation

Definition

The washing out of the bladder with sterile fluid through a urinary catheter.

Aims

1. To clear a blocked urinary catheter.
2. To remove blood clots or debris from the bladder which may lead to obstruction.
3. To instil drugs, such as antibacterial agents, into the bladder.
4. To prolong viability of a catheter in long-term catheterisation.

Assessment

Action	Rationale
Determine reason for and the type of bladder washout to be given (see Table 8.1).	To ensure appropriate preparation of patient and equipment.
Assess condition of patient.	To facilitate correct positioning without causing further discomfort.
	To ensure adequate explanation of procedure and reduce anxiety.

Planning

Equipment

    See Table 8.1.

Table 8.1 Types of bladder irrigation

Types of bladder irrigation	Indications for use	Equipment
Intermittent irrigation using a catheter-tipped syringe.	Postoperative prostatectomy irrigation without an indwelling 3-way catheter.	Bladder washout pack containing jug, receiver and waterproof sheet.
		Sterile disposable gloves.
		Warmed bottle of irrigation solution, usually normal saline 0.9%.
		Disposal bag.
		Sterile 60 ml catheter-tipped syringe.
		Sterile drainage bag and tubing.
		Alcohol-based swabs.
		Clamp, e.g. gate clip.
Irrigation using the sampling port of the drainage system and a syringe and needle.	For bladder irrigation or topical antibiotic treatment for patients with indwelling often long-standing closed system of urinary drainage and where breaking the circuit is contraindicated.	Warmed bottle/sachet of sterile irrigation fluid, e.g. normal saline 0.9%.
		Sterile gallipot.
		Sterile disposable gloves.
		Alcohol-based swabs.
		Clamp, e.g. gate clip.
		Sterile 50 ml syringe and appropriate size of needle.
Intermittent irrigation using prepacked sterile irrigatory solution.	For bladder irrigation with prepacked bactericidal agents. In patient with indwelling catheters requiring frequent irrigation to prevent infection and crystalisation.	Warmed plastic container of irrigatory solution, e.g. normal saline 0.9%.
		Sterile drainage bag and tubing.
		Sterile disposable gloves.
		Clamp, e.g. gate clip.
Continuous irrigation using a 3-way catheter.	Method of choice for immediate postoperative prostatectomy patients to prevent clot formation, assist drainage and facilitate haemostasis.	Sterile continuous irrigation set.
		Warmed sterile irrigation fluid, e.g. normal saline 0.9%.

Action	Rationale
Prepare appropriate equipment.	To reduce discomfort/shock to patient.
N.B. All irrigatory solutions should be given at body temperature. Solutions should be warmed, preferably in a heated storage cupboard. If no such cupboard is available, place irrigatory solution in sterile jug of warm water (approximately 40°C) and leave for 20 min. Dry bottle/sachets prior to use.	
Explain procedure to patient.	To ensure patient's consent and co-operation.
Position patient comfortably allowing easy access to catheter.	To maintain patient comfort and dignity.
Cleanse trolley.	To reduce risk of infection.
Assemble equipment on bottom shelf of trolley (see Wound Care procedure in Chapter 56).	To facilitate procedure.

Implementation

Intermittent irrigation using a catheter-tipped syringe

Action	Rationale
Wash hands using the Ayliffe Taylor technique and prepare the sterile field (see Wound Care procedure in Chapter 56).	To reduce risk of infection and to facilitate procedure.
Place water-repellent sheet and receiver underneath the catheter.	To protect bedclothes and to minimise the risk of infection.
Clamp catheter.	To prevent leakage on disconnecting catheter.
Disconnect catheter from drainage bag.	To facilitate procedure.

Discard drainage bag and tubing making a note of amount drained.	To prevent contamination and maintain the fluid output record.
Cleanse hands with alcohol hand rub.	To reduce risk of cross-infection.
Cleanse outside of catheter with alcohol-based swab and allow to dry for at least 90 seconds.	To reduce the risk of introducing infection through the catheter.
Wearing sterile gloves, fill the syringe with irrigating solution, expelling any air.	To prevent discomfort to the patient by the introduction of air into the bladder.
Release the clamp and inject the solution *slowly* via the catheter into the bladder.	To prevent the rapid injection of fluid which may cause discomfort to the patient.
Remove syringe and allow solution to drain back into the receiver.	This causes less discomfort to the patient than aspiration.
Apply gentle aspiration *only* if the fluid does not drain back freely.	To remove clots which could be causing an obstruction to the flow.
Estimate and ensure that the same quantity of fluid is returned each time.	Bladder distension may occur if the catheter is not draining freely.
Repeat procedure until there is evidence that the returning fluid is draining freely and contains no blood clots/debris.	To ensure that the bladder has been cleared of clots/debris and that there will be no obstruction to the drainage.
Connect the catheter to a sterile drainage bag immediately.	To reduce the risk of introducing infection into the catheter by closing the drainage system.
Measure the fluid contained in the receiver. The amount should equal or exceed the total amount of fluid used to perform the washout.	To confirm that all irrigation fluid has been returned.
Record observations of drainage in nursing records, e.g. clots, blood loss, etc.	To assist with the evaluation of care.

Intermittent irrigation using the sample port of the drainage system and a 50 ml syringe and needle

Action	Rationale
Ensure drainage bag is empty.	To facilitate accurate measurement of fluid returned.
Wash hands using the Ayliffe Taylor technique (see Wound Care procedure in Chapter 56).	To minimise risk of infection.
Prepare the sterile field.	To facilitate procedure.
Clamp catheter drainage tube below sample port.	To ensure fluid flows into bladder.
Clean sample port with alcohol-based swabs and allow to dry for a minimum of 90 seconds.	To reduce risk of infection.
Cleanse hands with alcohol hand rub.	To minimise risk of infection.
Wearing sterile gloves, draw irrigation solution into syringe.	To facilitate procedure.
Carefully puncture sample port.	To prevent injury to the nurse.
Gently introduce the prescribed amount of irrigatory fluid.	To minimise discomfort to the patient.
Ensure recommended waiting time is adhered to. Check manufacturer's/medical instructions.	To ensure optimum benefit from procedure.
Release clamp.	To allow drainage of irrigating fluid from bladder into drainage bag.
Empty drainage bag (see Emptying a Urine Drainage Bag procedure in Chapter 12).	To determine that the same quantity of fluid is returned.
Record the procedure and the result on appropriate nursing documentation.	To assist with the evaluation of care.

Intermittent irrigation using a pre-packed sterile irrigating fluid

Action	Rationale
Wash hands using the Ayliffe Taylor technique (see Wound Care procedure in Chapter 56).	To minimise the risk of infection.
Prepare sterile field (see Wound Care procedure in Chapter 56).	To facilitate procedure.
Place sterile waterproof sheet and receiver under catheter.	To receive leakage on disconnecting catheter.
Disconnect catheter from drainage bag and place in receiver.	To facilitate procedure.
Cleanse hands with alcohol hand rub and put on sterile gloves.	To reduce risk of introducing infection.
Remove cover from nozzle of pre-packed irrigating fluid and insert into end of catheter.	To facilitate procedure.
Allow solution to flow into the bladder, applying minimal pressure only.	To minimise discomfort to the patient.
Determine the patient's tolerance of the fluid.	Pre-packed solutions contain 100 ml and the patient may experience discomfort before total amount has been introduced.
Clamp the tube and allow prescribed waiting time. See manufacturer's/medical instructions.	To ensure optimum effect of procedure.
Release clamp.	To allow drainage of irrigating fluid from the bladder back into the bag.
Disconnect catheter from pre-packed solution and attach a sterile drainage bag immediately.	To reduce the risk of introducing infection via the catheter by closing the drainage system.
Measure fluid returned.	To determine that the same quantity of fluid is returned.

Record the procedure and the result on appropriate nursing documentation.	To assist in the evaluation of care.

Continuous bladder irrigation using three-way catheter

Action	**Rationale**
Wash hands using Ayliffe Taylor technique (see Wound Care procedure in Chapter 56).	To reduce the risk of infection.
Prepare sterile continuous irrigation set by priming the tubing.	To facilitate procedure.
Wearing sterile gloves, connect irrigation set to catheter.	To facilitate procedure and to prevent infection.
Allow fluid to flow at the prescribed rate (check medical instructions).	To ensure optimum effect of procedure.
Maintain careful observation of irrigation input and urinary output.	To detect fluid imbalance. To determine catheter patency.
Record observation of drainage and abnormalities, e.g. clots, in nursing records.	To assist in the evaluation of care.
Ensure adequate supply of warmed irrigation fluid is available.	Large quantities of fluid may be required for this procedure.
Once continuous irrigation has been discontinued, observe urine output for further haematuria which may necessitate recommencing bladder irrigation.	To prevent the complication of clot retention.

Evaluation

Potential problems of procedure	**Appropriate nursing action**
Retention of irrigation fluid.	The drainage system should be checked for faults, e.g. kinked tubing. A blocked catheter may require 'milking'.
	Inform medical staff.

Haemorrhage.	Inform medical staff.
Patient experiences severe pain during procedure.	The procedure should be discontinued and medical advice sought.
	Give analgesia as prescribed.
Infection.	Observe temperature of patient.
	Observe urine for signs of infection, e.g. cloudiness, offensive odour.
	Obtain a clean specimen of urine for culture.
	Inform medical staff.

Adaptations for home care

All working surfaces should be protected from drainage; likewise, the bed should be protected with plastic sheeting. A pair of Spencer Wells forceps may be used instead of a gate clip where specified. As bladder washouts are often given as an ongoing process for patients with long-standing urinary catheters, it is necessary that supplies of lotion/urotainers and equipment are regularly obtained. Relatives should, therefore, be advised on how prescriptions may be obtained.

References and further reading

Bard Limited (1985), *Guidelines for the Management of the Catheterised Patient.*
Gibson, T. (1980), 'Promoting a steady flow', *Nursing Mirror*, Supplement, 21 February.
Harper, W. (1981), 'An appraisal of 12 solutions used for bladder irrigation or instillation', *British Journal of Urology*, vol. 53, pp. 433–8.
James, J. (1984), 'Intermittent bladder irrigation', *Nursing Times*, Supplement, vol. 80(37).
Jenner, E. (1977), 'Specialised care – a closed system of urinary drainage', *Nursing Mirror*, Supplement, 3 November.
Kennedy, A. (1984), 'Trial of a new bladder washout system', *Nursing Times*, vol. 80(46), pp. 48–51.
Lawthian, P. (1988), 'Steps to combat infection', *Nursing Times*, vol. 84(12), pp. 64–6.

9   Taking and recording of blood pressure

Definition

To measure the force of blood exerted against the arterial walls to establish base-line values or detect deviations.

Assessment

Action	Rationale
Explain the procedure to the patient.	To allay fears and gain co-operation.
Select limb which is free from any form of injury/intravenous infusion.	To prevent discomfort to patient and to prevent disruption to circulation.
Check the baseline recording, if available.	To ensure that any difference in recordings is detected swiftly.
Check the frequency and timing of the recordings.	To ensure accurate monitoring.

Planning

Equipment

Sphygmomanometer with clearly visible meniscus.
Bladder of correct size.
Stethoscope.

Action	Rationale
Explain the procedure to the patient.	To gain co-operation.

Position patient comfortably. If lying or sitting, the patient should remain in the position for 3 min.

To enable correct measurement of blood pressure.

If standing, the patient should remain in the position for 1 min.

If sitting, place a pillow under the patient's arm.

To ensure comfort and reduce risk of arm movement which may interfere with recordings.

Measure cuff/bladder.

The correct sized cuff should be used or else recordings will be incorrect.

Remove clothing from limb where cuff is to be applied.

To prevent constriction of arm.

Implementation

Action

Rationale

Position forearm to be level with the heart.

If the arm is above heart level, blood pressure will be falsely low. If the arm is below heart level, blood pressure will be falsely high.

Position the centre of the bladder over the line of the artery 2–3 cm above the antecubital fossa.

The pressure when the cuff is inflated should be directly over the artery. The space of 2–3 cm allows room for stethoscope placement.

Secure cuff firmly.

A loose cuff leads to falsely high recordings.

Position arm slightly flexed at elbow. Support arm for patient or rest it on a surface.

If patient supports own arm, muscular contraction can raise diastolic pressure by as much as ten per cent.

Ensure cuff is at the level of the heart.

To ensure an accurate recording.

Place sphygmomanometer on a level surface at the eye level of the nurse.

To ensure an accurate recording.

Ensure mercury level is at zero.

To ensure an accurate recording.

Tighten thumbscrew on valve.	To prevent air escaping.
Locate brachial artery on antecubital space by feeling for pulse beat.	The branchial artery is superficial and can be easily palpated.
Inflate cuff for 3–5 seconds until pulsation disappears.	The point of disappearance represents the systolic pressure.
Deflate cuff slowly until you feel the pulse again.	
Place stethoscope lightly over the artery.	Pressure on the stethoscope or touching of cuff may grossly underestimate the diastolic pressure.
Inflate cuff again to 30 mm Hg above palpated systolic pressure.	
Deflate cuff slowly (2–3 mm Hg/seconds).	Rapid deflation may lead to faulty reading.
Note the level at which you hear two consecutive beats.	This is systolic pressure.
Continue to release until sounds disappear. Note reading.	Sounds disappear when blood flows easily in the artery. This is diastolic pressure.
Both pressures should be taken to the nearest 2 mm Hg.	To ensure accuracy.
Deflate cuff rapidly to zero.	
Remove cuff and record immediately on appropriate documentation.	Recording at completion of reading prevents error.

Evaluation

Potential problems of procedure	**Appropriate nursing action**
Muffled sounds persisting to zero point.	In adults this may indicate a medical condition.
	Report to the medical staff.

Faulty stethoscope or sphygmomanometer.

Check all equipment before use and ensure six monthly maintenance of sphygmomanometer.

Adaptation for home care

The procedure is carried out as described.

References and further reading

Bell, M. and Siklos, P. (1984), 'Recording blood pressure: accuracy of staff and equipment', *Nursing Times*, vol. 80(26), pp. 32–4.

Draper, P. (1987), 'Not a job for juniors', *Nursing Times*, vol. 83(10), pp. 58–62.

O'Brien, P. (1986), 'Recommendations on blood pressure measurement', *British Medical Journal*, vol. 293 (6547), pp. 611–15.

Quattrucci, J. (1977), 'The hygiene of stethoscopes', *Nursing Times*, February, pp. 193–5.

Rudy, S.F. (1986), 'Blood pressure techniques', *Nursing*, vol. 16(8), pp. 46–9.

Walker, M. (1984), 'Blood pressure recording I: Observation in the newly admitted patient', *Nursing Times*, vol. 80(26), pp. 28–32.

10   Blood transfusion

Definition

The administration.of whole blood or a component of blood directly into a vein.
N.B. This is a sterile procedure.

Assessment

See Intravenous Infusion procedure in Chapter 28.

Action	Rationale
Record the patient's temperature and pulse.	To provide a baseline on which to monitor any change in condition.
Check the efficiency of the established intravenous infusion.	To determine patency of cannula.
Check that normal saline 0.9 per cent is in use prior to the administration of blood.	To prevent haemolysis of the red cells.
Check that a giving set for the administration of blood is in use.	A blood filter is essential.

Planning

Equipment

See Intravenous Infusion procedure in Chapter 28.
Thermometer.
Temperature chart.
Giving set for the administration of blood.

Action	**Rationale**
Ensure collection of blood from the blood bank, allowing a minimum time of 15 min at room temperature prior to administration.	To prevent shock to the patient, due to the administration of cold blood.

Implementation

See Intraveneous Infusion procedure in Chapter 28.

Action	**Rationale**
Explain the procedure to the patient.	To gain consent for the transfusion of blood.
Check the unit of blood against the patient's records for correct: • Blood group • Rhesus factor • Serial number • Personal details • Hospital reference number.	To prevent misadministration of blood, this should be carried out by two nurses, one of whom is a registered nurse or in accordance with Health Authority policy.
Check the unit of blood to determine that it is within the expiry date.	To prevent misadministration of blood, this should be carried out by two nurses, one of whom is a registered nurse or in accordance with Health Authority policy.
Check the patient's identity bracelet against the unit of blood.	To prevent misadministration of blood, this should be carried out by two nurses, one of whom is a registered nurse or in accordance with Health Authority policy.
Replace the normal saline 0.9 per cent with the unit of blood.	
Reregulate blood flow (see Intravenous Infusion procedure in Chapter 28).	To ensure correct rate of flow.

Subtract the volume of the discarded normal saline 0.9 per cent.	To maintain an accurate record of fluid intake.
Record volume of blood and time of commencement of transfusion on the fluid balance chart.	To maintain an accurate record of transfused blood.
Record the patient's temperature and pulse hourly throughout the procedure.	To monitor for signs of reaction to the transfusion.

Evaluation

See also Intravenous Infusion procedure in Chapter 28.

Potential problems of procedure	Appropriate nursing action
A rise in temperature compared to the baseline observations.	Inform medical staff.
Anaphylactic shock.	Stop transfusion. Inform medical staff. Initiate resuscitation if necessary.
Loin pain, rigors and urticaria.	Stop infusion. Inform medical staff.
Rapid administration of large quantities of blood or blood transfusions to a patient with sickle cell anaemia.	A blood warmer should be used.
Blood not used within 1 hour of removal from the blood bank refrigerator.	Return blood to the blood bank for destruction. N.B. It must not be returned to the refrigerator for future use.

Adaptations for home care

This procedure is not applicable in the community.

References and further reading

Millam, D.A. (1988), 'Managing complications of intravenous therapy', *Nursing 88*, vol. 18(3), pp. 34–43.

Mintz, P.D. *et al.* (1986), 'The latest protocols for blood transfusion', *Nursing 86*, vol. 16(10), pp. 34–41.

Phillips, A. (1987), 'Are blood transfusions really safe?', *Nursing 87*, vol. 17(6), pp. 63–4.

Speechley, V. (1982), 'Intravenous therapy', *Nursing*, vol. 2(7), pp. 184–9.

Swaffield, L. (1987), 'Circulating the blood', *Nursing Times*, vol. 83(11), pp. 16–17.

11   Cardio-pulmonary resuscitation

Definition

Cardiac arrest

Cessation of the effective pumping action of the heart muscle.

Cardio-pulmonary resuscitation

The re-establishment of cardiac and pulmonary function by artificial means.

Assessment

Action	Rationale
Confirm cardiac/respiratory arrest by:	
• Observing the person's colour	
• Palpating the carotid or femoral pulse.	Absence of a major pulse indicates that the heart has stopped beating.
• Observing the respirations.	Breathing patterns may be absent or irregular.
• Assessing the level of consciousness.	Low cardiac output with poor tissue oxygenation will depress cerebral function.
• Checking pupil reaction.	Fixed, dilated pupils indicate cerebral anoxia.
• Observing colour of skin.	Signs of shock will be present and due to respiratory embarrassment, the patient might be cyanosed.

Planning

N.B. It is essential that all staff:

- Are aware of the location of the resuscitation equipment.
- Are familiar with the resuscitation procedure.
- Receive regular instruction from appropriate personnel.
- Check equipment daily or according to Health Authority policy.

Action	Rationale
Determine ratio of ventilation to cardiac compression to be adopted during the procedure by the operators, i.e. 1:5, 2:10, simultaneously.	To maximise efficiency and speed of procedure.

Equipment

Ambubag and selection of face masks.
Guedal airway.
Oxygen cylinder.   (if not piped to the bedside).
Suction apparatus.   (if not piped to the bedside).
Drug box.
Intubation equipment.
Equipment for intravenous infusion.
Defibrillator
Cardiac monitor

Implementation

Action	Rationale
On discovering a person in a collapsed state, summon help immediately and note the time.	To alert the medical staff and other relevant personnel. Cerebral oxygenation needs to be restored within 3 min to prevent irreversible brain damage.
Position patient supine on a firm surface, maintaining as much dignity as possible.	To ensure maximum effectiveness of the procedure. To reduce the distress of the other patients and any relatives present.

Remove secretions and/or loose-fitting dentures.	To reduce the risk of airway obstruction.
	N.B. Well-fitting dentures provide support and help obtain an airtight fit when a face mask is used.
Remove the head of the bed and/or any other obstruction.	To ensure easy access to the patient and to facilitate the procedure.
Hyperextend the neck and pull the lower jaw upwards.	To open the airway and prevent the tongue obstructing the airway.
Position the Guedal airway in the patient's mouth.	To prevent the tongue from obstructing the air passages.
Use the ambubag whenever possible in preference to mouth to mouth ventilation.	The operator does not come into contact with the patient's secretions, e.g. vomit or blood.
	It is less tiring for the operator.

Commence assisted ventilation

Using the ambubag

- Fit the mask of the ambubag snugly over the nose and mouth and compress the bag once.

This forces atmospheric air into the lungs.

N.B. The ambubag can be attached to the oxygen supply.

To provide more effective oxygenation.

Using mouth to mouth ventilation

- Pinch the patient's nose.

To ensure air is directed towards the lungs.

- Inhale deeply.

To ensure sufficient volume of air can be exhaled.

- Cover the patient's mouth with your own and exhale.

To force expired air into the lungs

N.B. For a patient with small features or a child, it may be necessary for the operator to cover the patient's nose and mouth to obtain maximum benefit.

Commence cardiac massage

This is done in conjunction with assisted ventilation.

• Clench the fist and sharply strike the lower third of the sternum once.	To stimulate the heart into action. Research is divided on the value of this aspect of the procedure.
• Place the heel of the hand over the lower third of patient's sternum and compress at the rate of one compression per second.	To reduce the risk of fracturing the ribs. To raise intrathoracic pressure, which is thought to squeeze blood into the lungs.
• Continue cardio-pulmonary resuscitation at the predetermined ratio until help arrives or spontaneous cardiac function returns.	To restore cerebral oxygenation.

Evaluation

It is essential during the cardio-pulmonary resuscitation to reassess every 60 seconds the patient's responsiveness to the procedure.

Potential problems of procedure	**Appropriate nursing action**
Potential patient awareness of procedure.	Give simple straightforward explanations throughout procedure.
Irreversible brain death.	Follow medical staff's instructions regarding termination of procedure.
Presence of the patient's relatives at the arrest.	Escort to appropriate waiting area and provide explanation and reassurance at the earliest opportunity.
Distress to other patients and their relatives when cardio-pulmonary function is not restored.	Provide explanation and support as soon as possible.
Staff distress.	Allow the opportunity to express feelings and emotions as necessary (see Last Offices procedure in Chapter 29).

Adaptations for home care

1. Summon help; dial 999 or, if possible, ask someone to do it for you.
2. Continue with procedure until ambulance arrives (nurse would not normally accompany patient to hospital).
3. Inform relatives/next of kin, as appropriate, of the situation.

References and further reading

Goodwin, R. (1988), 'Critical care: cardio-pulmonary resuscitation', *Nursing Times*, vol. 84(34), pp. 63–8.

Newbold, D. (1987) 'Critical care: the physiology of cardiac massage', *Nursing Times*, vol. 83(25), pp. 59–62.

Newbold, D. (1987), 'Critical care: external chest compression: the new skills', *Nursing Times*, vol. 83(26), pp. 41–3.

12   Catheter care

Definition

To insert a catheter into the bladder.

Reasons for procedure

1. To empty the bladder before and after some surgical procedures.
2. To relieve retention of urine.
3. To alleviate incontinence due to underlying medical condition.
4. To fill the bladder prior to ultrasound scan.
5. For accurate assessment of kidney function.

Aims

1. To cause as little psychological and physical trauma as possible.
2. To reduce the risk of infection.

Assessment

Action	Rationale
Determine specific/personal cultural requirements and ensure their fulfilment, e.g. request for female medical/nursing staff.	To gain patient's consent and co-operation and prevent personal or cultural offence.
Determine presence of any discharge/excreta requiring removal and cleansing prior to procedure.	To minimise the risk of infection.

Assess patient and choose correct size of catheter.

To prevent urethral trauma due to incorrect size of catheter.

N.B. Size 14 or 16 usual for an adult patient and balloon size 5–10 ml.

To prevent bladder spasm.

Planning

Equipment

One disposable plastic apron.
Cleaning solution, e.g. aqueous chlorhexidine 0.05 per cent (warmed sachets) in a clean bowl. Dry before use.
Two pairs of sterile gloves.
Correct type and size of catheter.
Adhesive strapping.
Catheter drainage bag.
Sterile water for injection.
10 ml syringe.
Adequate light source.
Alcohol hand rub.
Sterile kidney dish.
Two sterile gallipots.
Sterile green sheet to cover vulva.
Cotton wool balls.
One piece gauze.
Small nozzle.
One pair forceps.
Sterile lignocaine gel if required.
Disposal bag.
N.B. A catheterisation pack may be available containing some of the above equipment.

Action

Explain procedure.

Rationale

To minimise anxiety and to gain patient co-operation.

Obtain verbal consent for procedure.

To ensure the patient's full agreement to procedure.

Cleanse and prepare trolley (see Wound Care procedure in Chapter 56).

To facilitate procedure and reduce the risk of infection.

Implementation

Action	**Rationale**
Ensure patient dignity and privacy throughout procedure.	To minimise embarrassment.
Place patient in optimum position, usually dorsal with knees flexed apart.	Facilitates easy access to urethral and vulval area.
Reassure and observe patient throughout procedure.	To maintain co-operation and prevent sudden movement which may displace catheter.
Remove pad/catheter as appropriate.	
Wash hands, using Ayliffe Taylor technique (see Wound Care procedure in Chapter 56).	To prevent cross infection.
Using an aseptic technique, open packs and catheter covering. Wearing sterile gloves, lay out trolley.	To reduce the risk of infection.
Place sterile sheet over vulval area.	To prevent contamination from anal area and to create as clean an area as possible around the urethral orifice.
Clean vulval area from above downwards, swabbing each labia minora and finally urethral orifice.	To prevent contamination from anal area and to create as clean an area as possible around the urethral orifice.
Change gloves and place receiver between patient's legs.	To reduce the risk of infection.
Keeping labia open, insert catheter and drain residual urine into receiver.	

Catheter remaining *in situ*

Secure catheter in position by inflation of balloon with sterile water and use gentle traction to check catheter is in place.	To ensure retention of catheter.
Connect catheter to continuous drainage bag.	To reduce risk of infection by means of a closed drainage system.
Attach bag to recommended stand, ensuring a downward flow of urine.	To facilitate a flow of urine and to avoid backtracking of infection.

Secure catheter to inner thigh.	To prevent undue movement of catheter causing friction to urethra.
Dry perineum.	To promote patient comfort.
Reposition patient.	To promote patient comfort and dignity.
Dispose of used equipment and clear away trolley according to Health Authority policy.	To prevent cross-infection and trauma to staff.

N.B. Using clean gloves, it is recommended that the catheter is cleaned with soap and water on a twice-daily basis. If there is exudate present, an antiseptic solution may be used to clean the urethral orifice. A specimen of urine should be sent for culture and sensitivity.

Residual catheterisation

When urine ceases to flow withdraw catheter and discard.	
Dry vulva, perineum and buttocks if necessary.	To maintain patient comfort.
Reposition patient.	To maintain patient comfort.

Filling the bladder prior to ultrasound scan

Following insertion of catheter and cessation of urine flow, gently instil warmed sterile water (approximately 500 ml) via a syringe until patient complains of discomfort.	To facilitate accurate interpretation of scan.
Insert a sterile spigot into the end of the catheter.	To prevent leakage.

Evaluation

Potential problems of procedure	Appropriate nursing action
Shock due to rapid drainage of urine following severe distension.	Reduce rate of urine drainage by attaching a gate clip to catheter tubing to act as a regulator.

Contamination of catheter due to vaginal insertion.	Leave catheter in vaginal orifice, correctly identify urethral orifice and insert new sterile catheter, then remove vaginal catheter.
Urinary tract infection in patients with an indwelling catheter.	Use a closed drainage system. Encourage fluid intake. Perform catheter care as required. Avoid placing drainage bag above the level of the bladder to prevent backtracking of bacteria.
	Avoid catheter bag trailing on the floor.
	Use an appropriate stand.
	Emptying of bags should always be an aseptic procedure.
	Observe for signs of urinary tract infection.
Poor drainage.	Check patency of drainage system. Possible causes could be positioning of patient, affecting gravity of flow or incorrect stand for drainage bag.
Sore urethra.	Sterile lignocaine gel could be inserted.
Leaking past the catheter.	Investigate the cause. This may be due to an undersized catheter being inserted originally.

Catheter specimen of urine ▬▬▬▬▬▬▬▬▬▬▬▬

Definition

Collection of a sample of urine from a patient with an indwelling catheter.

Planning

Equipment

Gate clip/Spencer Wells clamp.
Sterile 10 ml syringe.

Alcohol-based swab.
Sterile needle – small diameter, e.g. 0.5 or 0.6 mm.
Universal container.
Clean gloves.

Action	Rationale
Explain reason and nature of procedure.	To minimise patient anxiety and gain patient co-operation.
Ensure privacy.	To minimise patient anxiety and gain patient co-operation.

Implementation

Action	Rationale
Apply a gate clip or appropriate clamp below the sample sleeve about 10 min before collecting the sample.	To enable an appropriate column of urine to accumulate in the drainage bag.
Wearing gloves, clean the sample sleeve present on catheter tubing with a swab. Allow to dry.	To create as clean an area as possible.
Using a syringe and needle at an angle of 45° draw off 10 ml of urine.	To avoid the nurse puncturing their finger with the needle.
Great care should be taken when inserting the needle into the sleeve.	To avoid the nurse puncturing their finger with the needle.
Remove gate clip.	To prevent obstruction to flow.
Place sample into universal container.	To facilitate immediate transfer to the laboratory and prevent contamination.
Dispose of used equipment according to Health Authority policy.	To prevent cross-infection and injury to staff.
Correctly label specimen.	To avoid unnecessary repetition of procedure and to facilitate quick receipt of results.

Evaluation

Potential problems of procedure	Appropriate nursing action
Insufficient urine present in catheter tubing.	Clamp tube below the sample sleeve until sufficient urine has been collected.
Specimen is required prior to commencement of antibiotics out of laboratory hours.	Store specimen at 4°C in specimen refrigerator.
Patient has commenced antibiotics before specimen is required.	Note the type of antibiotic on the pathology form.

Emptying of urine drainage bag ▬▬▬▬▬▬▬

Aims

1. To enable accurate measurement of urine/renal function at pre-stated times.
2. To prevent trauma to the neck of the bladder due to weight of drainage bag.

Assessment

Action	Rationale
Observe colour, amount and odour of urine. Report any abnormalities to medical staff.	To determine any abnormalities and facilitate prompt treatment.

Planning

Equipment

Clean gloves.
Designated alcohol spray.
Tissues.
Container – disposable urinal/bedpan preferred and paper cover.

Action	Rationale
Explain reason for and nature of procedure.	To minimise anxiety.

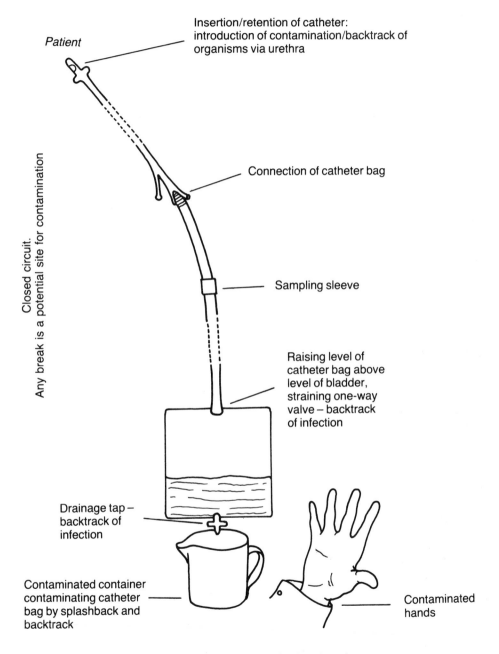

Figure 12.1 Possible sites of contamination of a catheter.

Implementation

Action	**Rationale**
Wearing gloves, spray outlet tap of catheter bag and allow to dry.	To reduce bacterial growth.
Drain urine into container.	
Using tissues, wipe away excess urine on the outlet tap. Respray tap and allow to dry.	To reduce bacterial growth and prevent backtracking of bacteria.
Measure and dispose of urine carefully.	To monitor fluid balance and prevent contamination.

Evaluation

Potential problems of procedure	**Appropriate nursing action**
Cross-infection.	Ensure procedure is always conducted as a sterile procedure.
Use of non-disposable jugs where there are no washing/disinfecting facilities may lead to cross-infection.	Use disposable or sterilised containers for collecting urine on every occasion.

Removal of self-retaining catheter

Assessment

Action	**Rationale**
Determine specific personal/cultural requests and ensure their fulfilment.	To gain patient's consent and co-operation and prevent personal or cultural offence.
Check urinary meatus for exudate. If exudate present cleansing is required prior to removal of catheter. (see Female Catheterisation procedure in this chapter).	To facilitate easier removal of catheter and to prepare the correct equipment.

Planning

Equipment

> Sterile disposable gloves.
> Syringe (check size required).
> Receiver.
> If cleansing is required:
>> Cotton wool balls
>> Gallipot
>> Antiseptic solution
>> Disposal bag.

Implementation

Action	**Rationale**
Place patient in the optimum position, usually dorsal.	To facilitate procedure.
Wearing gloves, clean around the catheter/meatal area if necessary.	To remove any exudate which may be present and prevent trauma when the catheter is removed.
Place receiver between the patient's legs.	To prevent soiling of sheets as catheter is removed.
Withdraw all the water from the catheter's balloon, using a syringe.	To avoid urethral trauma and to facilitate procedure.
Gently remove catheter and place into receiver.	
Reposition patient.	To promote patient comfort.
Dispose of used equipment according to Health Authority policy.	To prevent cross-infection and prevent injury to staff.

Evaluation

Potential problems of procedure	**Appropriate nursing action**
Patient's inability to pass urine following removal of catheter.	Monitor urinary output and observe for:

- Reduced volume of urine at each void.
- Patient discomfort.
- No urine has been voided for 8 hours.

If any of the above occur, inform medical staff.

Difficulty in removing a long-term catheter.

Inform medical staff.

Urinary tract infection following catheterisation.

Send first specimen voided for microbiological examination.

Adaptations for home care

1. The patient's bed should be protected with plastic sheeting.
2. All working surfaces should be protected from drainage.
3. A small torch may be necessary to ensure an adequate source of light.
4. On completion of the procedure, all equipment should be disposed of according to Health Authority policy.
5. All samples should be checked and patient/relatives should be advised regarding the obtaining of prescriptions for new catheters and drainage bags.
6. All catheter changes should be recorded on the patient's care plan and the date of the next visit agreed with the patient and relatives.

References and further reading

Ayliffe, G.A.J., Collins, B.J. and Taylor, L.J. (1982), *Hospital Acquired Infection – Principles and Prevention*, Wright & Sons, Bristol, pp. 41–4, 51–2.

Glenister, H. (1987), 'The passage of infection', *Nursing Times*, vol. 83(22), pp. 68–73.

Gooch, J. (1986), 'Catheter care', *The Professional Nurse*, vol. 1(8), pp. 207–8.

Jenner, E. (1983), 'Cutting the cost of catheter infections', *Nursing Times*, vol. 79(28), pp. 58–61.

13 Chest aspiration

Definition

To remove fluid from the pleural space for diagnostic or therapeutic purposes.

Assessment

Action	Rationale
Determine reason for procedure:	
• To remove pleural fluid.	To relieve respiratory embarrassment.
• To obtain specimen of fluid.	To assist diagnosis.
• To introduce drugs.	For therapeutic reasons.
	To ensure appropriate preparation of patient and equipment.
Assess condition of the patient.	To facilitate correct positioning of the patient.
	To determine the presence of a cough, when a linctus should be given prior to the procedure.
	To facilitate appropriate explanation of the procedure and to gain the patient's co-operation.

Planning

Equipment

Trolley.
Sterile dressing pack.

Sterile 500 ml jug.
10 ml syringe and assortment of needles.
Three-way tap.
Sterile tubing.
Antiseptic solution.
Local anaesthetic.
Sterile specimen pots.
Laboratory forms.
Disposal bag.
One pair sterile gloves.
Sterile paper towels.
Elastoplast/waterproof plaster.

Action	Rationale
Explain the procedure to the patient.	To obtain the co-operation and consent of the patient.
Position patient upright in bed or chair, leaning forward.	To aid breathing and to facilitate the accumulation of drainage in the base of the lung.
Position arms forward on to a firm surface.	To facilitate entry of needle by raising the scapula and opening the intercostal spaces.
Prepare trolley maintaining sterility.	To prevent infection.

Implementation

Action	Rationale
Remind the patient not to cough without warning.	To prevent the needle from puncturing the lung.
Observe vital signs during the procedure.	To detect respiratory distress, pain or shock.
Assist the doctor as required	To facilitate a safe procedure.
Ensure dressing is *in situ* on completion of procedure.	To protect wound site from contamination. To prevent staining of clothes.

Reposition patient in most comfortable position.	To facilitate breathing.
Dispose of equipment according to Health Authority policy.	To prevent injury to staff.

Evaluation

Potential problems of procedure	Appropriate nursing action
Respiratory embarrassment	Monitor vital signs of patient until condition is stable.
Reaction to intrapleural drugs.	Inform medical staff.

Adaptations for home care

This procedure is not applicable to the community.

References and further reading

Jamieson, E., McCall, J. and Blythe, R. (1988), *Guidelines for Clinical Nursing Practices*, Churchill Livingstone, Edinburgh, p. 132.

Pritchard, A.P. and Walker, V.A. (eds.) (1984), *The Royal Marsden Hospital Manual of Clinical Nursing Policies and Procedures*, Harper & Row, London, pp. 114–16.

14   Removal of sutures/clips

Definition

The removal of any non-absorbable material used to hold skin edges together.

Assessment

Action	Rationale
Assess the condition of the wound and degree of healing.	To prevent premature removal of sutures/clips.
Determine material to be removed.	To ensure appropriate equipment is assembled for use.
Determine the need for cleansing solution.	
N.B. Routine cleansing of clean/dry wound is unnecessary.	N.B. If wound is oozing and this requires cleansing, sterile gloves should be worn.

Planning

Equipment

> Appropriate dressing pack.
> Trolley.
> Cleansing solution (if necessary) at room temperature.
> Three sterile plastic gloves, if necessary.
> Alcohol hand rub.
> Adhesive tape.
> Appropriate sized dressing, if necessary.
> Disposal bag.

Sterile stitch or clip removers.
Any other specific equipment as required.

Action	**Rationale**
Select an appropriate environment.	To reduce the risk of cross-infection.
Wash hands thoroughly using the Ayliffe Taylor technique (see Wound Care procedure in Chapter 56)	To reduce the risk of cross-infection.
Cleanse the trolley according to Health Authority policy.	To reduce the risk of cross-infection.
Assemble the appropriate equipment on the bottom shelf of the trolley and attach disposal bag to the trolley.	To facilitate the dressing technique and reduce the risk of cross-infection.

Implementation

Action	**Rationale**
Explain the procedure to the patient.	To reduce anxiety and gain consent and co-operation.
Place the patient in an appropriate position and make them as comfortable as possible.	To ensure access to the site.
Wash hands thoroughly using Ayliffe Taylor technique or alcohol hand rub (See Wound Care procedure in Chapter 56).	To reduce the risk of cross-infection.
Open packs on to the top of the trolley and assemble equipment.	To ensure easy access to equipment.
Loosen and remove old dressing if present, using the adapted Hampshire Technique (see Wound Care procedure in Chapter 56).	To reduce the risk of contamination of hands.
Cleanse hands with alcohol hand rub.	To reduce the risk of cross-infection.

Wearing gloves and using the stitch cutter, remove sutures or, using clip remover, remove clips.

Cleanse wound if appropriate (see Wound Care procedure in Chapter 56).

Evaluation

Potential problems of procedure	Appropriate nursing action
Partial wound dehiscence.	Apply sterile towel soaked in warmed sterile normal saline.
	Inform nursing/medical staff.
Breakage of suture material on removal.	Attempt to remove remaining fragment.
	If unsuccessful, document appropriately and inform nursing/ medical staff.

Adaptations for home care

See Wound Care procedure in Chapter 56.

References and further reading

See Wound Care – Chapter 56.

15   Principles of caring for the confused patient

Definition

The term confusion is used to describe a state of perplexity, muddled thought processes and disorientation. Confusion is a misleading term, because it is vague and covers a variety of symptoms and behaviour.

1. *Objective confusion* is a term used to describe a state of confusion which is obvious to the outsider, e.g. brain damage.
2. *Subjective confusion* is a term used when patients complain of feeling disorganised, forgetful and aimless, e.g. bereavement, anxiety states.
3. *Acute confusion* is sudden and severe in onset due to the toxic effects of drugs, disease or disorders, e.g. constipation, alcohol, infections or metabolic imbalance.
4. *Chronic confusion* has an insidious onset and is usually progressive, e.g. long-term effect of metabolic disorders, use and abuse of drugs and dementia.

Aim

To protect the patient from harm and to maximise their contact with reality.

Assessment

The patient who is confused may exhibit some of the following characteristics:

1. *Disorientation* – this may be to time, place or person.
2. *Impaired Consciousness* – may occur after anaesthesia, administration of drugs, following head injury or trauma.
3. *Altered Facial Expression* – perplexed, bewildered, distressed, anxious.
4. *Impaired Intellectual Function* – impaired judgement and/or memory. Difficulty in following simple instructions.
5. *Changes in Usual Behaviour* – loss of inhibitions, uncharacteristic verbal responses, aggressive outbursts. See Care for the Potentially Violent Patient in Chapter 55.

Planning

Communication will be easier and more effective if:

Action	Rationale
Allowance is made for any sensory deprivation – check if patient usually wears spectacles or a hearing aid.	Optimum functioning of the sensory organs will help the communication process.
Words are pronounced clearly and slowly. Requests or instructions are made as simple as possible.	Simple requests or instructions are easier to follow and understand.
Ideally one or two nurses attend to the patient.	Constant changes in staff will increase disorientation.
Even if it appears that the patient does not understand what is happening, always explain every procedure and activity.	Sudden, unexplained changes are frightening and unsettling. The patient may understand more than they appear to.

Implementation

Action	Rationale
Avoid changes in ward and bed allocation.	Familiar surroundings promote feelings of security and reduce disorientation.
Encourage the use of personal possessions.	To promote independence, self-identity, dignity and reduce disorientation.
Identify and maintain the patient's own routine. Be as consistent as possible in your approach.	To minimise disorientation.
Allow time for dressing and other activities.	The patient may complete the task if given a little more time. This will promote independence and increase self-esteem.

Ensure a safe environment without restricting independence.	To promote independence and maintain patient safety.
Remind patient by gentle conversation of basic information, e.g. your name, their name, which meal is next.	To maximise contact with reality.
Avoid talking down to the patient. Always refer to them by their preferred name or correct title if unable to indicate otherwise.	To show respect and maintain dignity.
Do not talk about patient as if they were not present.	To enhance patient's self-esteem and reduce feelings of helplessness.

Evaluation

Potential problems of procedure **Appropriate nursing action**

Confusion can be associated with violent aggression.	See Care of the Potentially Violent Patient in Chapter 55.
Tendency to wander.	Ensure nursing staff are aware and that the patient is wearing an identity band.
Antisocial behaviour.	Protect other patients.
	Attempt to re-educate patient.
	Adopt a consistent approach by all members of staff.

Adaptations for home care

The principles of the above procedure can be used within the community setting.

References and further reading

Joseph, C. (1983), 'The confused elderly patient', *Modern Medicine*, vol. 28, no. 23, pp. 26–35.
Millard, P. (1978), 'Rehabilitate or to vegetate', *Nursing Mirror*, 16 March, pp. 14–6.
Sugden, J. and Saxby, P.J. (1985), 'The confused elderly patient', *Nursing*, 2nd series (the add-on journal of *Clinical Nursing*), vol. 2(35), pp. 1022–5.

16 Prevention of cross-infection

Definition

Infection is the result of the deposition and multiplication of organisms within the body, causing disease. Cross-infection is the spread of organisms from one person to another, directly or indirectly, either by the airborne or contact route.

Aim

To prevent cross-infection by removing the source/reservoir, blocking route of spread and/or enhancing the individual's resistance to infection.

Assessment

Action	Rationale
Determine the source and potential route of infection.	To facilitate implementation of infection control policies.
Determine individuals at risk.	To facilitate implementation of infection control policies.

Planning

Action	Rationale
Determine precautions to be taken by referring to Table 16.1 provided or Health Authority infection control policy.	To prevent cross-infection.
Assemble appropriate equipment.	To prevent cross-infection.

Table 16.1 Source of infection

Necessary precautions	Wound	Skin	Secretion	Blood	Enteric	Respiratory	Protective isolation
Single room	Desirable	Necessary, door shut	Desirable	Desirable	Desirable	Necessary, door shut	Necessary, door shut
Apron to be worn	Handling wound/dressings	Patient contact	Handling secretions/patient contact	Handling blood/body fluids	Handling excreta/soiled bed linen	Handling secretions/contaminated articles	Patient contact
Mask to be worn	No	No	No	No	No	No	Not usually necessary
Routine hand wash	Before and after contact with site and immediate environment			After contact with blood/body fluids	After contact with faeces	After contact with sputum	Before and after patient contact
Gloves to be worn	Contact with infected area or dressing			Handling blood/body fluids	Handling contaminated articles		Not usually necessary
Nursing equipment	Disposable, disinfect or sterilise				Own labelled bedpan, commode		Disinfect/sterilise before use

Table 16.1 (Cont.)

Necessary precautions	Wound	Skin	Secretion	Blood	Enteric	Respiratory	Protective isolation
Crockery/cutlery		Normal ward issue			Disposable[1]		Normal ward issue
Linen[4]	Normal disposal[2]			Appropriate linen bags			Normal disposal
Rubbish[4]				Appropriate plastic bags			Normal disposal
Disinfectant[5]		Clear soluble phenolic		Hypochlorite		Clear soluble phenolic[3]	
Comments							Exclude staff/visitors with known infections

[1] Unless central wash up available
[2] Unless otherwise advised
[3] Unless hepatitis A, then hypochlorite
[4] Refer to Health Authority clinical waste disposal policy/laundry policy
[5] Refer to Health Authority disinfection policy

Disease	Isolation precautions
AIDS	Blood, secretion/excretion (body fluids)
Anthrax, cutaneous	Wound
Anthrax, pulmonary	Respiratory
Brucellosis	None
Chicken pox	Respiratory
Cholera	Enteric
Diphtheria	Respiratory
Dysentery	Enteric
Food poisoning	Enteric
Gastroenteritis	Enteric
Hepatitis A	Enteric
Hepatitis B	Blood
Hepatitis non-A non-B	Blood
Legionnaire's disease	None
Leptospirosis	Secretion/excretion (urine)
Leprosy	Secretion/excretion (nasal discharge)
Lice	Skin
Malaria	None
Measles	Respiratory
Meningitis, meningococcal	Secretion/excretion (nasal discharge)
Meningitis, viral	None
Ophthalmia neonatorum	Secretion/excretion
Plague	secretion excretion (bubo aspirate)
Poliomyelitis, acute	Respiratory, enteric
Psittacosis	Respiratory
Rabies	Secretion/excretion (saliva)
Relapsing fever	Skin (prior to delousing)
Ringworm	Skin
Rubella	Respiratory
Scabies	Skin
Shingles	Secretion/excretion (lesion discharge)
Staphylococcal disease	Respiratory, skin or wound (as appropriate)
Streptococcal disease	Respiratory, skin or secretion/excretion (All maternity and scarlet fever or cutaneous)
Tetanus	None
TB, open pulmonary	Respiratory
TB, non-respiratory	Secretion/excretion (depends on site)
Typhoid	Enteric, secretion/excretion (urine)
Typhus	Skin
Viral haemorrhagic fever	Seek advice from control of infection nurse/doctor
Whooping cough	Respiratory
Yellow fever	Blood, secretion/excretion (urine)

Source: Central Birmingham Health Authority Control of Infection Policy.

Figure 16.1 Source isolation categories.

Seek appropriate advice from infection control officer.	To prevent cross-infection.
Explain any precautions to the patient and relatives.	To gain co-operation and reduce anxiety.

Implementation

Care for infected patient according to Figure 16.1.	To facilitate safe nursing practice and prevent cross-infection.

Evaluation

Potential problem of procedure	**Appropriate nursing action**
An outbreak of infection occurs or continues to spread.	Inform infection control officer.
	Methods of preventing spread must be reviewed by infection control team.

Adaptations for home care

The principles of the above procedures could be applied in the community.

References and further reading

Acquired Infection in the N.H.S. and its Prevention, (1978), Royal College of Nursing.

Ayliffe, G.A.J., Collins, B.J. and Taylor, L.J. (1982), *Hospital Acquired Infection – Principles and Prevention*, Wright & Sons, Bristol.

Bagshawe, K.D. (1978), 'Isolating patients in hospital to control infection', *British Medical Journal*, vol. 2, pp. 609–12.

Central Birmingham Health Authority Control of Infection Policy.

Central Birmingham Health Authority Disinfectant and Antiseptic Policy.

Lowbury, E.J.L., Ayliffe, G.A.J., Geddes, A.M. and Williams, J.D. (1981), *Control of Hospital Infection*, 2nd edn, Chapman & Hall, London.

Maurer, I.M. (1985), *Hospital Hygiene*, 3rd edn, Edward Arnold, London.

17 Principles of caring for the depressed patient

Definition

Depression is a disturbance of mood characterised by an overwhelming feeling of sadness, unworthiness, guilt and low self-esteem. N.B. This procedure should be read in conjunction with the procedure for Principles of Caring for the Suicidal Patient in Chapter 48.

Assessment

Many different types of behaviour are associated with depression. The primary indicator in any assessment is that the patient's usual pattern of behaviour and emotional responses have changed. Changes associated with depression are as follows:

1. Apparent sadness – despondency, despair; more than just a passing phase of low spirits, it shows in speech, facial expression and posture.
2. Reported sadness – reports of depressed mood which may not show in appearance, feelings of being beyond help and without hope.
3. Inner tension – anxiety, tension, dread.
4. Reduced sleep – changes in sleep pattern; patient does not feel refreshed on waking.
5. Altered appetite pattern.
6. Constipation.
7. Concentration difficulties – difficulty organising thoughts and concentrating.
8. Lethargy – no 'get up and go', difficulty in performing everyday activities.
9. Agitation – inability to relax.
10. Changes in emotional response – reduced interest in surrounding activities that normally give pleasure; inability to show usual emotional response to people or circumstances.
11. Pessimistic thoughts – only negative about the future, guilt feelings, sense of remorse and ruin.
12. Suicidal thoughts – feeling that life is not worthwhile, suicidal thoughts and plans.

Implementation

Action	Rationale
Promote optimum physical health by:	
• Observing patient's food and fluid intake.	The patient may not be aware of or interested in their own physical needs.
• Recording input, output and weight.	
• Observing bowel habits.	
• Determining the patient's likes and dislikes regarding diet and provide an acceptable diet in small, well-presented portions.	To monitor the patient's nutritional state.
• Offering nutritional supplements as appropriate.	
• Avoiding reference to not eating as a cause of ill-health.	The patient may wish to die.
Provide an environment conducive to sleep at night.	Limiting disturbance and providing comfort will promote sleep.
Set agreed limits on the amount of time that the patient can spend in bed. Avoid allowing sleep during the day.	A good balance of rest and exercise will help the patient sleep better and encourage the patient to socialise with others.
Provide a safe environment.	The physical safety of the patient is a priority.
Maintain the patient's contact with reality by orientating patient to person, time and place.	To decrease disorientation and hallucinations or delusions.
Establish a relationship of trust.	The patient's ability and motivation to interact with others may be impaired.
Increase the patient's self-esteem by:	
• Promoting good personal hygiene.	Patients with low esteem may be unaware of their personal hygiene.
• Providing simple activities that can be accomplished.	Positive encouragement and achievement will enhance self-esteem.
• Giving praise and encouragement.	Positive encouragement and achievement will enhance self-esteem.

Encourage the patient to express his/her feelings.	Expression of feelings will help relieve despair or sadness.

Evaluation

Regular evaluation of the patient is essential to monitor for improvement and to detect a deterioration in the patient's mental and physical state at the earliest opportunity.

Potential problems of procedure	Appropriate nursing action
Risk of suicide.	Follow procedure for the Principles of Caring for the Suicidal Patient in Chapter 48.
Anxious relatives. N.B. Caring for the depressed patient over a period of time is extremely stressful.	Provide support, reassurance and information.

Adaptations for home care

The principles of the above procedure may be adapted for use within the community setting.

References and further reading

Montgomery, S.A. and Asbery, M. (1979), 'A new depression scale designed to be sensitive to change', *British Journal of Psychiatry*, vol. 134, pp. 382–9.
Schultz, J.M. and Dark, S. (1986), *Manual of Psychiatric Nursing Care Plans*, Little, Brown & Co., Boston.
Stuart, G.W. and Sundeen, S.J. (1983), *The Principles and Practice of Psychiatric Nursing*, 2nd edn, C.V. Mosby, St Louis, Miss.

18   Discharge from hospital

Definition

The termination of a patient's stay in hospital and transference home or to another institution. N.B. Most people are eager to go home from hospital, although others, due to their infirmity or condition may be transferred to another institution or have to live with others. To them, discharge is an anxious time.

Aim

To provide the relevant information and support and/or equipment, drugs and treatment, to enable the patient to resume as independent a life as possible.

Assessment

Action	Rationale
Commence preparation for discharge as soon as the patient is admitted to hospital in consultation with patient, relatives and professionals.	This ensures all types of help can be arranged.
Determine skills that require to be taught.	
All skills taught to patients and relatives need to be supervised and practised under supervision before discharge, taking into account their knowledge and capabilities.	To ensure all skills are carried out safely.

Communicating

Question	Action	Rationale
Are there any language difficulties?	Identify interpreter.	To facilitate communication and reduce frustration.
Are there any speech difficulties?	Contact speech therapist for advice and/or therapy.	To improve communication.
Are there any hearing difficulties?	Refer to appropriate personnel, e.g. Audiometry Department and/or British Telecom (see number for Careline in directory).	To facilitate communication.
Are the next of kin involved in the discharge procedure?	Contact and discuss discharge arrangements.	To find the best solution for any problems and facilitate co-operation.
Following discharge what professional links are required?	Identify and/or contact relevant personnel, e.g. GP, stoma therapist, social worker.	To give support facilitating recovery.
What voluntary organisations may be able to help?	Give name and address of appropriate organisation (see references).	

Breathing

Question	Action	Rationale
Is teaching and/or equipment required for nebulisers, inhalers, oxygen or tracheostomy care?	Teach and supervise patient and/or relatives the relevant skills. Order equipment needed.	To ensure patients and/or relatives are proficient and safe and that treatment is continued.

Does the patient smoke?	Advise on individual's health and, when oxygen in use, the environmental hazard.	To increase patient's knowledge. To maintain safety.

Maintaining safe environment

Is there sufficient family support at home? Is the home suitable for the patient's needs?	Contact appropriate community personnel involved, e.g. primary health care team medical social worker, liaison nurse.	To facilitate a home assessment to be undertaken and to effect a smooth discharge from hospital.
Is there a wound which requires a dressing?	Ensure patient has sufficient dressings for immediate needs, according to Health Authority policy.	To ensure continuity of care.
Is medication required to continue after discharge?	Teach dosage, route and side effects to patient and relatives as appropriate. Inform how to obtain further supplies if necessary.	To continue treatment and reduce risk of over or underdosing.

Eating and drinking

Are there any ongoing problems?	Contact relevant personnel, e.g. dietician, occupational therapist.	To maintain independence and ensure adequate and appropriate nutrition and hydration.

Washing, dressing and eliminating

Are there any ongoing problems?	Contact relevant personnel, e.g. continence adviser, primary health care team, stoma therapist, occupational therapist.	To maintain independence.

Mobilising

Are walking aids required?	Contact physiotherapist (N.B. when a walking frame or wheelchair is required at home, extra space needs to be ordered in ambulance or hospital car for discharge).	To maintain independence. To facilitate discharge.
Is hospital transport necessary?	Order transport in advance, according to Health Authority policy.	If relatives are unable to assist.
Is follow up physiotherapy required?	Ensure appointment and transport is arranged.	To continue treatment.

Sleeping and resting

Is specific night care needed?	Liaise with night carers.	Some patients demonstrate different behaviour at night.
Is specific advice necessary to prevent or minimise recurrence or exacerbation of the condition?	Education of patient and relatives accordingly.	To prevent further problems occurring.

Maintaining body temperature

Is the patient at risk of hypothermia?	Refer to medical social worker.	To reduce risk of hypothermia.

Expressing sexuality

Is advice on resumption of sexual activity required?, e.g. after hysterectomy, myocardial infarction or hip replacement.	Advise accordingly.	The patient is sometimes too embarrassed to ask.

Working and playing

Is advice on self-certification or medical certificate required?	Advise accordingly.	Continuity of salary or supplementary benefit.
Is support needed re: returning to work, loss of work or learning new skills?	Contact relevant personnel e.g. medical social worker, employment rehabilitation officer.	To reduce anxiety.

Dying

Is specialist help and/or information required?	Contact relevant personnel, e.g. hospice team, primary health care team, MacMillan Nursing Service.	To facilitate patient's and relatives' preference and to provide support.

Planning

Action	**Rationale**
Work in conjunction with all personnel involved with patient, giving sufficient time.	To avoid confusion and disappointment.
Ensure key, food, warmth in home are available on discharge. Refer to a check-list pertinent to clinical area.	Reduce risk of unnecessary readmission. To ensure all aspects of discharge are considered.

Implementation

Action	**Rationale**
Use appropriate documents and link personnel to contact primary health care team.	To minimise mistakes.
Should drugs need to be administered by community nurses, ensure written instructions are given by medical staff.	To meet legal requirement.

If patient's self-discharge is taken against medical advice, contact medical officer.	To meet legal requirements.
Complete relevant documents and note in nursing records.	
Order equipment in advance with a discharge date in view.	To allow time for delivery.
Teach appropriate skills – see Assessment in this chapter.	Maintains safety and reduces anxiety.
Ensure patient is still fit for discharge on day of departure.	Prevents unnecessary readmission to hospital and patient distress.
Give out-patient appointment if required and arrange transport if necessary.	To maintain continuity of care.
Ensure patient has: • Dressings. • A letter for primary health care team. • Drugs. • Property and valuables. N.B. If valuables are in hospital safe, may need time for their collection (see Health Authority policy). • Ensure patient is safely conveyed to transport.	Prevents distress and ensures a smooth discharge.

Evaluation

Potential problems of procedure	**Appropriate nursing action**
Failure to be discharged as planned.	Contact all relevant personnel and inform of change of plans.
Unexpected change of discharge address.	Contact all relevant personnel and inform of change of plans.

Relevance of all planned arrangements may change.	Reassess immediately prior to discharge to avoid wasted time.
Patients with, or in contact with, resistant organisms, e.g. methicillin-resistant Staphylococcus aureus.	Refer to infection control guidelines of the Health Authority or seek advice from the infection control officer.

Adaptations for home care

This procedure is not applicable to the community.

References and further reading

Bowling, A. and Betts, G. (1984), 'From hospital to home 2 – communication on discharge', *Nursing Times*, vol. 80(32), pp. 33.

Bowling, A. and Betts, G. (1984), 'From hospital to home 5 – communication on discharge', *Nursing Times*, vol. 80(33), pp. 44–6.

Clay, T. (1984), 'From hospital to home – divide and rule?', *Nursing Times*, vol. 81(10), pp. 48–9.

Department of Health and Social Security Circular (1989), *Discharge of Patients From Hospital*, HC(89)5.

Gibb, S. (1985), 'From hospital to home – the yellow one is my water pill', *Nursing Times*, vol. 81(9), pp. 29–30.

Heyward Jones, I. (1987, 1988), 'Helping hands – an information directory' *Nursing Times*, monthly instalments, February 1987 to April 1988.

Jupp, M. and Sims, S. (1986), 'Discharge planning – going home', *Nursing Times*, vol. 82(40), pp. 40–2.

Kemp, J. (1985), 'Discharge planning, it's different at night', *Geriatric Nursing*, vol. 5(5), pp. 20–2.

Potterton, D. (1984), 'From hospital to home 3 – the yawning gap', *Nursing Times*, vol. 80(32), pp. 34–5.

Price, B. (1984), 'From hospital to home 1 – a framework for patient education', *Nursing Times*, vol. 80(32), pp. 28–30.

Sines, D. (1984), 'From hospital to home 4 – change for the better?', *Nursing Times*, vol. 80(33), pp. 42–4.

Vaughan, B.F. and Taylor, K. (1988), 'Discharge procedures – homeward bound', *Nursing Times*, vol. 84(15), pp. 28–31.

19 Administration of an enema or suppository

Definition

An enema is a liquid for insertion into the rectum which is either absorbed or ejected. A suppository is a medication incorporated in a fatty or glycogelatin base that is administered rectally and melts at body temperature.

It is the responsibility of the medical staff to determine the need for and to prescribe, the relevant enema or suppository.

Types

1. Retention enema, e.g. arachis oil, used to soften faeces and facilitate relief of chronic constipation or for the topical administration of drugs, e.g. steroids.
2. Evacuant enema, e.g. docusate sodium used to promote defaecation in acute constipation or to clear the bowel prior to surgery or radiological examination.
3. Therapeutic suppositories, e.g. aminophylline.
4. Evacuant suppositories, e.g. glycerol used to soften faeces and facilitate defaecation.

Assessment

Action	Rationale
Determine the patient's ability to lie on the left side.	For anatomical ease of administration.
Ascertain what specific toilet needs are required, e.g. commode or bedpan.	To reduce anxiety and avoid unnecessary embarrassment.
Determine the patient's ability to understand and/or carry out instructions.	To facilitate patient's co-operation.

| Ascertain that the patient's bladder is empty and, prior to drug administration, their bowels also. | To prevent rapid return of enema/suppository. |

Planning

Equipment

Protective covering for bed, e.g. incontinence pad, plastic sheet and draw sheet.
Appropriate covering for patient.
Prescribed enema (warmed if advised) or suppositories plus appropriate lubricant.
Disposable apron (for nurse).
Disposable gloves (for nurse).
Commode or bedpan.
Tissues/toilet roll.
Disposal bag.

Action	**Rationale**
Explain procedure to patient and ensure privacy.	To reduce embarrassment and anxiety.
Obtain verbal consent.	To gain patient's co-operation

Implementation

Action	**Rationale**
Turn patient to left side with knees drawn up and buttocks to edge of bed.	For ease of administration.
Protect bed.	To absorb leakages and prevent skin discomfort.
Advise patient to retain enema or suppository for as long as possible.	To maximise effect.
N.B. Suppositories for evacuant use should be used rounded end first.	Stimulates and irritates rectum for faecal expulsion.
Suppositories used for drug administration should be given blunt end first.	Reduces irritation of rectum and facilitates drug absorption.

After administration, make patient comfortable with call bell and/or toilet facility close to hand.	To reduce anxiety.
Inspect result for volume and consistency.	To evaluate result.
Ensure hand washing facility for both patient and nurse is provided.	To facilitate hygiene standards.
Record result on relevant documents.	To maintain accurate records.

Evaluation

Potential problems of procedure	Appropriate nursing action
Poor result of evacuant enema or suppository.	Repeat procedure, following advice from nurse in charge or medical staff.
Drugs returned.	Check with medical staff before further administration, checking patient's rectum prior to procedure.
Pain during procedure.	Stop procedure, comfort patient, inform medical staff.
Pain during defaecation.	Comfort patient and refer to nurse in charge or medical staff.
Incorrect lubricant to glycerol suppositories.	Dip suppositories in warm water only, as other lubricants inhibit hydroscopic action.
Inability of patient to assume left lateral position.	Right lateral, prone and supine positions can be used with great care.

Adaptations for home care

1. Ensure electric blanket has been removed from bed before commencing procedure.
2. Ensure adequate protection for working surface, furniture and carpet.
3. Provide container for used equipment.
4. In event of poor hand-washing facilities, an alcohol-based hand rub may be used.

References and further reading

Booth, S. and Booth, B. (1986), 'Aperients can be deceptive', *Nursing Times*, vol. 82(39), pp. 38–9.

Brier, L.J. (1986), 'Eliminating suppositories in bowel training', *American Journal of Nursing*, vol. 86(5), pp. 522–4.

Duffin, H.M., Castleden, C.M. and Chaudhry, A.Y. (1981), 'Are enemas necessary?', *Nursing Times*, vol. 77(45), pp. 1940–1.

Ractoo, S. and Baumber, C.D. (1983), 'Testing times', *Nursing Mirror*, vol. 156(24), pp. 26–7.

Smith, S. (1984), 'Constipation (1). A beginner's guide to research', *Nursing Times*, vol. 80(22), pp. 64–7.

Walker, R. (1982), 'Suppository insertion', *World Medicine*, vol. 18(5), p. 58.

Wright, D. (1984), 'Constipation (2). The researchers' view', *Nursing Times*, vol. 80(22), pp. 65–7.

20   Enteral feeding

Definition

The administration of required nutrients, into the gastro-intestinal tract via a route other than oral. These routes may be:

> Naso-gastric.
> Naso-duodenal/jejunal.
> Gastrostomy, a feeding tube directly into the stomach via the abdominal wall inserted as a surgical procedure.
> Jejunostomy, a feeding tube directly into the jejunum via the abdominal wall inserted as a surgical procedure.

Assessment

Action	Rationale
Determine route of administration.	To select appropriate equipment.
Determine method of administration.	To select appropriate equipment.

Planning

Equipment

> Fine-bore feeding tube.
> Reservoir container.
> Enteral giving set.
> Adhesive tape.
> Mobile stand.
> Feed – as prescribed by dietitian (should be at room temperature).
> Enteral feeding pump, if appropriate.

Action	Rationale
Select an appropriate environment with the necessary equipment.	To ensure privacy and allow opportunity for discussion.

Implementation

Action	Rationale
Explain the procedure.	To gain consent and co-operation.
Check the tube is correctly positioned (see Naso-gastric Intubation procedure in Chapter 32).	To ensure safe delivery of feed.
Wash hands.	To reduce the risk of cross-infection in an already weakened patient.
Assemble the equipment.	To ensure safe and efficient delivery of feed.
Check the feed.	To ensure correct feed is given at the correct temperature.
Commence feed, check all connections are secure to maintain closed delivery system.	To reduce the risk of contamination.

Evaluation

Potential problems of procedure	Appropriate nursing action
Nausea.	Reduce the flow rate.
	Seek nursing/medical advice.
Vomiting.	Stop the feed.
	Seek nursing/medical advice.
Diarrhoea.	Reduce delivery rate of the feed.
	Ensure that the feed is at room temperature.
	Seek nursing/medical advice.
	Save specimen feed and stool.

Tube blocked.	Aspirate. If no aspirate, seek nursing/medical advice.
Excoriation of skin around gastrostomy or jejunostomy site.	Protect the skin appropriately.

N.B. The feed should not be used for longer than the recommended time expiry limit. If feeds are decanted into a reservoir for any reason, care must be taken not to contaminate them.

Adaptations for home care

When patients are discharged from hospital, it is the responsibility of the staff to ensure adequate information is given to the patient and community staff regarding the feed and the equipment required.

References and further reading

Bastow, M., Greaves, P. and Allison, S. (1982), 'Microbial contamination of enteral feeds', *Human Nutrition, Applied Nutrition*, vol. 36A, pp. 213–17.

Grant, A. and Todd, E. (1987), *Enteral and Parenteral Nutrition*, vol. 2, Blackwell, Oxford.

Phillips, G.D. and Odgers, C.L. (1986), *Parenteral and Enteral Nutrition – a practical guide*, 3rd edn, Churchill Livingstone, Edinburgh.

21 Eye care

Eye bathing ━━━━━━━━━━━━━━━━━━━━━━━━━━━━━━━

Definition

Bathing the eyes with a solution to remove discharge or secretions.

Assessment

Action	Rationale
Assess the eye for: • Swelling. • Inflammation. • Discharge.	To determine need for procedure and to assist with planning.
Determine presence of pain.	May indicate the need for medical intervention.
Determine the presence of any bruising.	To avoid further trauma or pain during procedure.

Planning

Equipment

    Sterile eye pack containing:
      lint/soft gauze
      paper towel
      gallipot.
    Lotion, e.g. normal saline.
    Disposal bag.

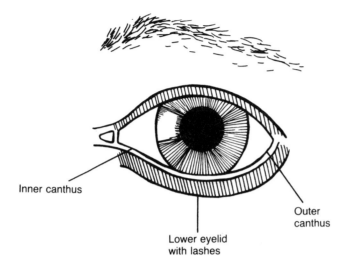

Inner canthus

Outer canthus

Lower eyelid
with lashes

Figure 21.1 The inner and the outer canthus of an eye.

N.B. A clean pack should be used for each procedure and each eye. Cotton wool should not be used, as this may leave strands across the eye.

Implementation

Action	**Rationale**
Explain procedure to patient.	To obtain consent and co-operation and to reduce anxiety.
Select optimum position, usually head tilted back and well supported.	To discourage patient from moving during the procedure and to maintain comfort.
Ensure adequate light.	To enable the nurse to see the eyes clearly.
Swab lids from inner to outer canthus.	To reduce the spread of any existing infection and to avoid corneal abrasion.
Use a clean swab each time, until all discharge has been removed.	
Dry the area.	To discourage bacterial growth.

Evaluation

Potential problems of procedure	Appropriate nursing action
Excessive discharge	Refer for medical opinion.
	Swab for culture and sensitivity as subsequent antibiotic therapy may be required.
Excessive discomfort.	Refer for medical opinion.
	Swab for culture and sensitivity as subsequent antibiotic therapy may be required.

Adaptions for home care

This procedure is carried out as described, using every opportunity to teach both patient and relative.

Instilling eye drops or ointment ▬▬▬▬▬▬▬

Definition

The application of eye drops or ointment for diagnostic or therapeutic reasons.

Assessment

Action	Rationale
Determine the condition of the eye/eyes.	To assess the need for bathing prior to procedure (see Eye Bathing procedure in this chapter).

Planning

Equipment

      Prescribed eye drops/ointment.
      Paper tissues.
      Patient's prescription sheet.

Action	Rationale
Check drops/ointment against prescription sheet according to hospital policy	To ensure that drops/ointment are instilled as prescribed (see Oral Drug Administration procedure in Chapter 36).

Check expiry date	To ensure medication is viable.

N.B. Individual drops/ointment should be prescribed for each patient and each eye treated separately.

Implementation

Action	**Rationale**
Explain procedure to the patient.	To obtain consent and co-operation and to reduce anxiety.
Select optimum position, usually head tilted back and well supported.	To discourage patient from moving during the procedure and to maintain comfort.
Check patient according to hospital policy.	To ensure correct patient.
Ask patient to look upwards and, using tissue, slightly invert lower lid.	To ensure the drops or ointment are instilled in the correct place.
Place a drop in the centre of lower fornix.	To facilitate maximum retention of solution.
Ask patient to gently close the eye after instillation of drop.	To disperse the solution across the eye.
Repeat as prescribed.	
Ointment should be applied from inner to outer canthus.	To ensure correct application and to minimise risk of infection.
Use a tissue to dry surrounding area.	To promote patient comfort.
Teach procedure to patient as appropriate.	To enable subsequent self-administration.
Store drops/ointment as recommended.	To maintain viability.

N.B. Antibiotics may be kept in the fridge.

Evaluation

Potential problems of procedure	Appropriate nursing action
Blurred vision, due to the application of ointment or mydriatic drops.	Advise patient not to drive, if relevant.
Allergic reactions to prescribed ointment/drops.	Inform medical staff and discontinue use.

Adaptation for home care

Patient or relative should be taught to undertake this procedure.

Irrigation of the eye ▬▬▬▬▬▬▬▬▬▬▬▬▬▬▬▬

Definition

The process of washing out the eye with a continuous flow of water or medicated solution.

Aims

1. To remove foreign matter, i.e. glass, dust.
2. To alleviate the effect of irritant fumes.
3. To counteract the effects of chemicals.

Assessment

Action	Rationale
Determine the reason for the procedure.	To establish whether the irrigation is needed.

N.B. The patient's verbal account of the incident is imperative as there may be no evidence when observing the eyes to suggest an injury has occurred.

Planning

Equipment

Sterile gauze squares.
Receiver.
Sterile undine.
Protective waterproof sheet.
Lotion, e.g. normal saline.
A phosphate buffer may be used for burns.

Implementation

Action	Rationale
Explain procedure to the patient.	To obtain co-operation and consent and to relieve anxiety.
Fill undine with solution, which should be warmed.	To promote patient comfort.
Select optimum position, usually head well-supported and tilted back, inclined towards the affected eye.	To facilitate procedure and prevent contamination of the other eye.
Cover the patient's chest and shoulders with waterproof sheet.	To protect clothing.
Instruct patient to hold receiver against their cheek.	To collect drainage.
Pour a small amount of solution over the back of the hand.	To ensure correct temperature of the fluid, i.e. body temperature.
Gently pour a small amount of the irrigating solution onto the patient's cheek.	To adjust patient to the feel of the solution.
Ask patient to look up, pull down the lower lid and irrigate from inner to outer canthus along the lower fornix.	To maximise the effect of the procedure and to disperse irrigation fluid across the eye.
Ask patient to look down, raise upper lid and irrigate from inner to outer canthus.	To maximise the effect of the procedure.

N.B. Irrigation should continue for at least 5–10 min.

Dry surrounding area.	To promote patient comfort.
Refer to casualty officer.	To determine the need for further treatment.

Evaluation

Potential problems of procedure	**Appropriate nursing action**
Extreme pain due to sensitivity of cornea.	Avoid unnecessary light.
	Apply eye pad.
	Reassure patient.
	Inform medical staff.

Adaptation for home care

This procedure is not applicable to the community.

References and further reading

Grimstone, D. (1986), 'Nursing care of the eye', *Occupational Health*, vol. 38(4), pp. 115–20.
Nelson, J. and Kopietz, L. (1987), 'Chemical injuries to the eyes: emergency, intermediate and long term care', *Post Graduate Medicine*, Occular Burns, vol. 81(4), pp. 62–75.

22 Gastric washout

Definition

Irrigation of the stomach to remove contents. N.B. This procedure is normally carried out by the medical staff, assisted by trained nursing staff.

Assessment

Action	Rationale
Determine reason for procedure, e.g. ingestion of harmful substances.	The procedure would not be undertaken if corrosives had been ingested, to reduce risk of further damage.
Determine whether the patient is conscious or unconscious.	Unconscious patients must be intubated prior to the procedure, to reduce the risk of aspiration.
Determine approximate time of ingestion.	
N.B. The procedure may be carried out within 24 hours of ingestion (this should be assessed by the medical staff)	To enable contents to be assessed and sent for further investigation (aspirate may be kept for up to two weeks).

Planning

Equipment

Wide bore gastric tubing.
Funnel.
Jug.

Solution as prescribed.
Bucket.
Guedal airway.
Clamp.
Plastic apron.
Plastic sheet.
Lubrication.
Suction apparatus.
50 ml syringe with catheter mount connection.
Receiver.
Blue litmus paper.
Tissues.
Disposal bag.
Emergency resuscitation equipment.

Action	**Rationale**
A hard-based trolley with tilts should be used.	To enable resuscitation, if necessary.
Select an appropriate area, usually a side room, with all the necessary equipment.	To ensure privacy for the patient, during a distressing procedure.
Ensure the emergency equipment is available.	Vagal stimulation may induce cardiac arrest.

Implementation

Action	**Rationale**
Explain the procedure to the patient.	To gain patient's co-operation and attempt to reduce anxiety.
Select an appropriate position for the patient, usually the left lateral position.	To maintain a clear airway and facilitate stomach drainage.
Remove false teeth and any debris from the patient's mouth.	To reduce the risk of inhalation.
Pass the lubricated wide-bore gastric tube via the mouth into the stomach.	To ease the passage of the tube.

Aspirate and test the stomach contents with the blue litmus paper.	To confirm that the tube is in the stomach; the litmus paper should turn pink.
Ensure a specimen is collected, if requested.	To send for laboratory analysis.
Test the temperature of the solution, which should be tepid.	To prevent sudden lowering of body temperature.
Inject between 100 and 500 ml of prescribed solution at any one time into the stomach.	To ensure solution reaches all areas of the stomach.
Record total volume given.	To monitor that the volume given is returned.
Syphon washout contents from the stomach back into the bucket.	To allow close observation of the contents and volume.
Repeat the procedure until contents clear.	
Clamp the tube and withdraw quickly.	To prevent inhalation and aspiration of any fluid.
Position the patient appropriately.	To reduce the risk of aspiration.
Observe patient closely.	To reduce anxiety, allow early detection of any change in condition and maintain patient safety.

Evaluation

Potential problems of procedure	Appropriate nursing action
Blood in the washout contents.	Medical staff must be informed.
Lowered body temperature.	Ensure warm environment.

This procedure may be carried out prior to surgery, as prescribed by medical staff. A Ryles tube passed naso-gastrically and 50 ml syringe, would be used (see also Naso-gastric Intubation procedure in Chapter 32).

Adaptations for home care

This procedure would not be conducted in the community.

References and further reading

Jamieson, E., McCall, J. and Blythe, R. (1988), *Guidelines for Clinical Nursing Practices*, Churchill Livingstone, Edinburgh.

23   High vaginal swab

Definition

To obtain a specimen from high inside the vagina for diagnostic purposes.

Assessment

Action	**Rationale**
Determine specific personal/cultural requests and ensure their fulfilment.	To gain patient's consent and co-operation and prevent personal and cultural offence.
Determine presence of vaginal discharge.	To assess the amount, colour and odour of vaginal discharge/blood.

Planning

Equipment

    Disposable gloves.
    Sterile swab with glass sleeve and protective cover.
    Clean pad.

Action	**Rationale**
Explain reason and nature of procedure.	To minimise anxiety and to promote patient co-operation.
Obtain verbal consent for procedure.	To ensure the patient's full agreement to the procedure.

Implementation

Action	Rationale
Ensure patient dignity and privacy throughout procedure.	To minimise embarrassment.
Place patient in optimum position, usually dorsal with knees flexed apart.	To facilitate procedure.
Wearing gloves, remove protective cover of swab.	To prevent cross-infection.
Gently insert glass tube containing sterile swab high into the vagina.	To prevent contamination of swab during insertion.
Pass swab through the glass sleeve.	To obtain specimen.
Withdraw swab into glass sleeve and return to protective cover.	To prevent contamination of swab during removal and transportation and to prevent cross-infection.
Apply clean pad and reposition patient.	To promote patient hygiene and comfort.
Clearly label specimen container.	To ensure the correct result is obtained and to prevent unnecessary repetition of procedure.

Evaluation

Potential problems of procedure	Appropriate nursing action
Loss of viability of organisms as swab dries.	Send specimen to the laboratory promptly. If delay is expected a transport medium should be used.

Adaptations for home care

This procedure may be conducted as described in the community.

References and further reading

Reynolds, M. (1984), *Gynaecological Nursing*, Blackwell Scientific Publications, Oxford, pp. 30–3.

Pritchard, A.P. and Walker, V.A. (eds.) (1984), *The Royal Marsden Hospital Manual of Clinical Nursing Policies and Procedures*, Harper & Row, London, p. 378.

24   Inhalation

Definition

The breathing in of steam and/or vapourised medicated solution.

Aims

1. To loosen secretions in the respiratory tract and aid expectoration of sputum.
2. To reduce the risk of secretions building up in vulnerable patients.

Assessment

Action	Rationale
Assess the mental and physical ability of the patient to manage the procedure.	To prevent injury from scalding or ingesting the substance.

Planning

Equipment

Nelson inhaler with rubber bung.
Appropriate solution, e.g. tincture of benzoin.
Boiling water.
Bowl to contain inhaler.
Padding, e.g. towel.
Suitable glass or plastic mouthpiece.
Gauze and tape.
Sputum pot and tissues.
Disposal bag.

Action	**Rationale**
Ensure sensitive approach to procedure	Promote patient dignity and well-being of others.
Avoid meal times.	
Explain the procedure.	To gain co-operation and facilitate inhalation.
Position the patient upright, preferably in a chair.	To ensure stability of inhalation equipment.
Place a table in front of the patient.	To ensure stability of inhalation equipment.
Prepare the patient as required.	To ensure patient safety.
Ensure bung is secure.	To ensure patient safety.
Protect the mouth piece with gauze and secure with tape.	To ensure patient safety.
Ensure air inlet faces away from the patient.	To ensure patient safety.
Secure the inhaler into the outer bowl with the padding.	To ensure patient safety.

Implementation

Action	**Rationale**
Ensure patient closes lips over the mouthpiece and inhales deeply through the mouth.	To maximise the effect of the procedure.
Ensure patient exhales into general atmosphere.	To prevent scalding the patient by displacement of the solution.
Remove inhaler when the fluid has cooled.	As the procedure is no longer effective.

Evaluation

This procedure should be evaluated for effectiveness. Criteria for monitoring effectiveness of procedure should include observation of sputum for amount/ viscosity/colour and patient assessment of effectiveness, e.g. relief of pain. Evaluation of effectiveness of procedure should be noted in the patient's nursing records.

Adaptations for home care

A narrow jug may be supplemented with caution if a Nelson inhaler is not available.

References and further reading

Jamieson, E., McCall, J. and Blythe, R. (1988), *Guidelines for Clinical Nursing Practices*, Churchill Livingstone, Edinburgh, p. 98.

25   Injections

Definition

The administration of drugs directly into body tissue using a syringe and hollow needle.

Methods of administration

Intradermal

Fluid administered under the skin which raises a wheal, e.g. Mantoux tests. A maximum of 0.5 ml can be given by this route.

Subcutaneous

Fluid administered into the connective tissue layer beneath the skin, e.g. insulin. A maximum of 2 ml can be given by this route.

Intramuscular

Fluid administered into the muscle layer. A maximum of 5 ml can be given via this route.

Z. Track

Fluid administered into the muscle layer after the skin is retracted from the entry site prior to the insertion of the needle and released following removal of needle, e.g. iron, to prevent staining of skin.

Assessment

Action	Rationale
Determine the reason for the injection and seek the patient's consent.	To facilitate treatment, gain patient's co-operation and reduce anxiety.

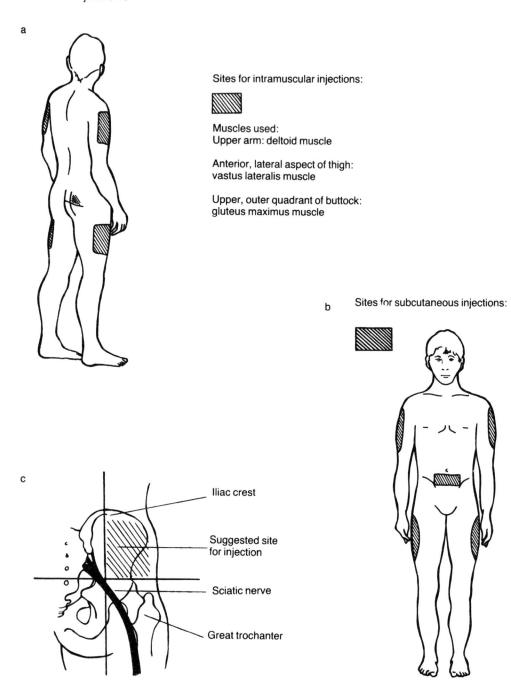

a

Sites for intramuscular injections:

Muscles used:
Upper arm: deltoid muscle

Anterior, lateral aspect of thigh:
vastus lateralis muscle

Upper, outer quadrant of buttock:
gluteus maximus muscle

b   Sites for subcutaneous injections:

c

Iliac crest

Suggested site
for injection

Sciatic nerve

Great trochanter

Figure 25.1 Sites for intramuscular and subcutaneous injections.

Table 25.1 Types of injection with related equipment and anatomical sites

Type of injection	Specific equipment	Preferred site of administration	Angle of needle	Anatomical position
Intramuscular	Appropriate sized syringe according to amount of fluid to be given. 40 mm needle.	Quadriceps muscle: lateral mid third of thigh. Gluteal muscle: upper outer quadrant of buttock. N.B. Position must be checked by trained member of staff due to proximity of sciatic nerve. Deltoid muscle: upper arm.	90°	See Figure 25.1.
Subcutaneous	2 ml syringe. 25 mm needle.	Outer surface of upper arm. Abdomen. Lateral mid third of thigh.	45° Some prepacked syringes with an integral needle may have alternative instructions, e.g. give at 90° angle. Please follow manufacturer's instructions.	See Figure 25.1.
Intradermal	1 ml syringe. 16 mm needle.	Inner surfaces of the forearm.	10°	See Figure 25.1.
Z track	As intramuscular injection	Preferably gluteal muscle.	90°	See Figure 25.1.

From prescription sheet determine:

- The drug.
- The dose.
- The route.
- The specified times of administration.
- Doctor's signature and date.

To assemble the correct equipment and determine the appropriate site (see Figure 25.1 and Table 25.1).

Planning

Equipment

Prescription sheet.
Receiver.
Alcohol-based swab (two, if a bottle with a rubber seal is used).
Appropriate syringe and needle.
Prescribed drug.
Sterile solvent for injection, if the drug to be used is in powder form.
Plastic ampoule cap or nursing towel.
File.
Dry cotton wool swab.

Implementation

Action	**Rationale**
Prepare the syringe and needle, leaving needle cover in place for as long as possible.	To maintain asepsis and safety.
Draw up solution.	

Using single dose ampoule

Shake down any liquid from ampoule top.	To ensure the full dose is given.
Determine whether ampoule is pre-stressed. If not, score neck with a file.	To facilitate opening of ampoule.
Warm ampoule in hand for 30 seconds.	To prevent glass particles entering solution for injection.
	N.B. Warmth causes an over-pressure which prevents ingression of glass particles on snapping the ampoule.
Protect top of ampoule with plastic cap or, in the absence of a plastic cap, use a folded paper towel.	To prevent injury to the nurse. *Care should always be taken.*

Using both hands, snap open ampoule and draw fluid into syringe.	To prevent injury to the nurse. Care should be always be taken.
Dispose of ampoule according to Health Authority policy.	To prevent injury to staff

Using multidose vial

Clean the rubber seal of bottle with alcohol-impregnated swab and allow to dry.	To ensure asepsis.
Inject air, equal to the amount of medication to be withdrawn, into the bottle.	To facilitate easy aspiration of solution.
Aspirate appropriate amount of solution into syringe.	
Expel air from the syringe after replacing the needle cap.	To prevent the introduction of air emboli and to prevent medication being sprayed into the atmosphere.

Determine whether or not to change the needle.

N.B. The needle should be changed in the following circumstances:

• When using a bottle with a rubber seal.	Needle may be blunted or contaminated by particles of rubber.
• When using viscous fluid.	The needle becomes coated with the solution.
• When using a preparation which may stain the skin.	The needle becomes coated with the solution.
• If the needle is blunted by hitting the side or bottom of the ampoule.	To prevent unnecessary pain to the patient.
• If the needle is contaminated.	To prevent introduction of infection.
Take the prescription sheet, swab and loaded syringe in a receiver to the patient.	To facilitate procedure.
Check identity of patient against the prescription sheet (see Oral Drug	To prevent misadministration of drug.

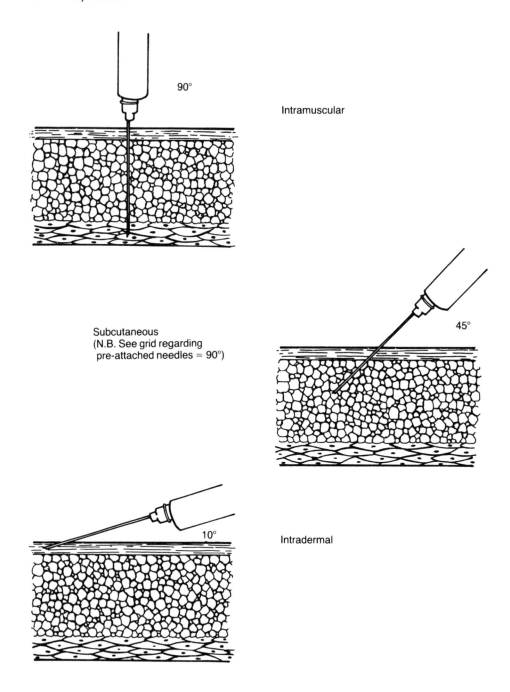

90°

Intramuscular

Subcutaneous
(N.B. See grid regarding
 pre-attached needles = 90°)

45°

10°   Intradermal

Figure 25.2 Angles for insertion of needle (see Table 25.1).

Administration procedure in Chapter 36).

Explain the procedure and position patient appropriately, ensuring privacy.	To facilitate procedure and reduce anxiety.
Insert needle (see Figure 25.2 and Table 25.1).	
N.B. Swabbing with an alcohol-based swab is not normally required prior to subcutaneous, intramuscular or intradermal injections.	Research has demonstrated that this fulfils no aseptic purpose where the skin is physically clean.
Prior to intravenous injections, swabbing is still recommended but must be allowed to dry (i.e. a minimum of 90 seconds).	
Withdraw plunger.	To confirm that needle has not penetrated a blood vessel. If blood present, withdraw and insert needle again.
Administer solution and withdraw needle.	
Reposition patient.	To ensure patient comfort.
Record administration of drug on appropriate documents.	To provide an accurate record.
Discard needles and syringe into designated rigid container (see Health Authority policy).	To prevent injury to staff.
N.B. It is essential that needles remain unsheathed and connected to syringe prior to immediate disposal into rigid container.	To prevent injury to staff.

Evaluation

Potential problems of procedure	Appropriate nursing action
Hitting bone.	Withdraw needle slightly prior to administration of fluid.
Administering solutions that stain the skin, e.g. iron.	Z. tracking should reduce this considerably (see Table 25.1).
Leakage of fluid from injection site.	Apply gentle pressure with sterile dressing swab.
Persistent pain following injection.	Inform medical staff.
Viscous substances for administration, e.g. ACTH	Give slowly to prevent build up of pressure.

Adaptations for home care

The community nurse should always carry adrenalin together with administration instructions for use in the event of a severe allergic reaction.

Planning

Prepare a suitable working surface using a paper towel to provide a clean area. Carry out any prescribed instructions/observations prior to administration of the drug.

Evaluation

Advise patient/carer of:

- The safe storage of the drug, e.g. out of reach of children.
- The safe disposal of obsolete drugs or drugs no longer required in accordance with Health Authority policy.
- When and how to get further prescriptions from the general practitioner.

References and further reading

Keen, M.F. (1986), 'Comparison of intramuscular injection techniques to reduce site discomfort and lesions', *Nursing Research*, vol. 35, no. 4.

26   Intrapleural drainage

Definition

An underwater seal system of drainage that prevents air entering into the pleural or mediastinal space.

Insertion of drain ▬▬▬▬▬▬▬▬▬▬▬▬▬▬▬▬▬▬▬▬

Assessment

Action	Rationale
Assess condition of the patient.	To facilitate correct positioning of the patient.
	To facilitate appropriate explanation and to gain the patient's co-operation.

Planning

Equipment

    Dressing pack.
    Paper towels.
    Chest drain and trocar.
    Assorted handles and blades.
    Artery and sinus forceps
    2/0 mersilk on a hand-held cutting needle.
    Antiseptic lotion.
    Local anaesthetic.
    Keyhole dressing.
    Adhesive dressing.
    Chest drainage bottle and tubing.
    Bottle stand.

Sterile normal saline.
Two chest drain clamps
Sterile gloves.
Disposal bag.
Appropriate chest radiographs.

Action	Rationale
Expain the procedure to the patient.	To obtain consent and co-operation of patient.
Prepare trolley, maintaining sterility.	To prevent infection.
Prepare bottle with sterile normal saline to calibrated level.	To ensure underwater seal.
Position patient upright in bed, leaning forward, arms forward on to a firm surface.	To aid patient comfort and breathing and facilitate entry of trocar.

Implementation

Action	Rationale
Assist the doctor as required.	
Attach tube to long drain of the bottle.	To ensure correct functioning of underwater seal system.
Check oscillation of fluid within the tubing of the bottle on inspiration and expiration.	To determine expansion of lung and patency of tube.
Ensure keyhole dressing around tube is *in situ*.	To protect wound site from contamination.
Ensure long drainage tube is approximately 2 cm below fluid level.	Too high – seal may be broken. Too low – a greater intrapleural pressure is required to expel air/fluid.
Attach short tube to suction apparatus (if ordered), at a prescribed pressure.	To aid drainage.
Observe and comfort patient throughout the procedure.	To detect increased respiratory distress and shock.
Reposition patient.	To facilitate drainage and promote patient comfort.

Support tubing.	To prevent dislodging and kinking of tubing.
	To prevent reflux of fluid into pleural space.
	To promote patient comfort.
Record the original fluid level on chest drain chart.	To ensure accurate measurement of drainage.

Evaluation

Potential problems of procedure	Appropriate nursing action
Excessive bubbling.	Check drainage system is patent.
	Inform medical staff.
	If drainage system is intact, an antifoam agent may be used to counteract excessive bubbling and enable the nurse to assess accurate drainage.
Aspiration of drainage fluid into the pleural space.	Ensure bottle is never lifted above level of patient's waist.
Disconnection of tubing, resulting in the entry of air into the pleural space.	Clamps should be easily accessible by the bedside for use in accidental disconnection and when changing the bottle.
Unnecessary clamping of drainage tube resulting in increased intrapleural pressure.	Clamping of tube is only necessary in accidental disconnection and when changing the bottle.

Caring for the patient with intrapleural drainage ▬▬▬▬

Implementation

Action	Rationale
Encourage patient to breathe deeply and cough.	To promote drainage and aid reinflation of lung.

Encourage patient to mobilise.	To promote drainage.
Milk tubing only if required.	To ensure patency of tube and to prevent clot formation.

Changing of underwater seal bottle ▬▬▬▬▬▬▬

Planning

Equipment

Sterile drainage bottle.
Sterile normal saline.
Two pairs chest drain clamps.
Sterile disposable gloves.

Action	**Rationale**
Explain the procedure to the patient.	To allay fear.
Prepare bottle with sterile saline to calibrated level, maintaining sterility.	To identify correct drainage total and prevent infection.

Implementation

This is a sterile procedure (see Wound Care procedure in Chapter 56).

Action	**Rationale**
Clamp tubing with two pairs of chest drain clamps as near to the chest wall as possible.	To prevent air entering the pleural space when underwater seal is broken.
Change bottle as quickly as possible and remove clamps.	To avoid increased intrapleural pressure.
Check oscillation of fluid level.	To determine patency of system.
Note change of bottle and fluid level on chart.	To allow accurate record of drainage.
Dispose of equipment according to Health Authority policy.	To prevent infection/injury to staff.

Removal of intrapleural drains ▬▬▬▬▬▬▬▬▬▬▬▬▬

Planning

Equipment

> Dressing pack.
> Stitch cutter.
> Sterile paraffin gauze squares.
> Dressing pad.
> Sterile paper towels.
> Adhesive tape.
> Sterile disposable gloves.

Action	Rationale
Explain the procedure to the patient.	To gain co-operation and consent.
Explain the need to take a deep breath and hold whilst tube is removed.	To prevent pneumothorax.
Prepare trolley, maintaining sterility.	To prevent infection.

Implementation

To promote speed and safety this procedure should be carried out by two nurses working in unison.

Action	Rationale
Conduct procedure maintaining sterility (see Wound Care procedure in Chapter 56).	To prevent infection.
Differentiate the purse string suture.	To facilitate closure of the wound as the tube is removed.
Differentiate and cut the suture holding the tube *in situ*.	To allow removal of tube.
Instruct patient to hold their breath as the tube is removed.	To minimise the risk of tension pneumothorax.
Pull purse string together and tie as the tube is removed.	To close wound and prevent air entering the pleural/mediastinal cavity.

Instruct patient to breathe out
normally, following closure of wound.

Cover wound with dry dressing.   To prevent contamination.

Reposition patient.   To promote comfort.

Dispose of equipment according to   To maintain staff safety.
Health Authority policy.

Evaluation

Potential problems of procedure   **Appropriate nursing action**

The purse strings may snap.   Apply a pad of paraffin gauze to help
                                              seal the hole and cover with an
                                              occlusive dressing.

The hole may not close adequately.   Apply a pad of paraffin gauze to help
                                              seal the hole and cover with an
                                              occlusive dressing.

To patient may develop acute   Sit patient up, well-supported, and
dyspnoea.   inform medical staff immediately.

Adaptations for home care

This procedure is not applicable in the community.

References and further reading

Carroll, P.F. (1986), 'The ins and outs of chest drainage systems', *Nursing*, vol. 16(12),
    pp. 26–34.
Duncan, C.R. and Erickson, R.S. (1982), 'Pressure associated with chest tube stripping',
    Heart & Lung, vol. 11(2), pp. 166–71.
Duncan, C.R., Erickson., R.S. and Weigal, R.M. (1987), 'Effects of chest tube management
    on drainage after cardiac surgery', *Heart & Lung*, vol. 16(1), pp. 1–9.
Erickson, R.S. (1981), 'Chest tubes – they're really not that complicated', *Nursing*, vol.
    11(5), pp. 34–43.
Erickson, R.S. (1981), 'Solving chest tube problems', *Nursing*, vol. 11(6), pp. 62–8.
Quinn, A. (1986), 'Thora drain III – closed chest drainage made simpler and safer', *Nursing*,
    vol. 16(9), pp. 46–51.

27   Intravenous bolus injection

Definition

The administration of drugs directly into a vein using a pre-sited cannula. N.B. This is an extended role procedure which requires a certificate of competence for the accountable nurse (refer to Health Authority policy):

- It is the medical staff's responsibility to administer the first dose, except in designated areas.
- Two nurses, an accountable nurse and one other, are required to check the preparation and the administration of the drug, to ensure safe practice.
- Prepared intravenous drugs must be given immediately. Never prepare more than one patient's medication at a time.

This procedure must be used in conjunction with the Health Authority's policy for the prescribing, handling, custody and administration of drugs.

Assessment

Action	Rationale
Determine from the patient's prescription sheet:	To ensure safe delivery of the prescribed drug.
<ul><li>Any known allergies.</li><li>The drug.</li><li>The dose.</li><li>The route.</li><li>The specified times of administration.</li><li>Valid medical signature.</li></ul>	
Determine the patient's condition.	To establish the patient's suitability to receive the drug.

Check cannula site.   To detect any signs of inflammation
                                       and extravasation.

Planning

Equipment

Tray/receiver.
Prescription sheet.
Alcohol spray or swab (two swabs if a bottle with a rubber seal is used).
Two syringes of appropriate size.
Two needles of appropriate size.
Prescribed drugs.
Sterile water for injections or specified diluent, if the drug to be used is in
    powder form (see manufacturer's instructions).
For flushing, use 2 ml sodium chloride 0.9 per cent for injection (1 ml to
    ensure patency, 1 ml after administration).
This flushing solution need not be prescribed on the treatment sheet.
If a flushing solution other than sodium chloride 0.9 per cent is used, it must
    be prescribed by a medical officer.

Implementation

Action   **Rationale**

Explain procedure to the patient and   To gain patient's consent and co-
the reason for giving the drug.   operation.

Draw up solutions.

Using a single dose ampoule

Shake down any liquid from ampoule   To ensure the full dose is given.
top.

Determine whether ampoule is pre-   To facilitate safe opening of the
stressed. If not, score ampoule neck   ampoule.
using a clean file.

Protect top of ampoule with approved   To prevent injury to nurse.
ampoule opener, plastic cap or, in the
absence of an opener, use a folded   Care should always be taken.
paper towel.

Snap open ampoule and draw fluid
into syringe.

Dispose of ampoule according to
Health Authority policy.

To prevent injury to staff.

Using a vial

Clean the rubber seal of bottle with
alcohol-based swab/spray and allow to
dry.

To ensure asepsis.

When reconstituting a powder, add
appropriate solvent as stated in
manufacturer's instructions.

To ensure safe delivery of medication.

When powder has dissolved, inject air
into the bottle equal to the amount of
medication to be withdrawn.

To ensure safe delivery of medication.

Aspirate appropriate amount of
solution into syringe.

To ensure safe delivery of medication.

Dilute further to comply with
manufacturer's instructions.

To ensure safe delivery of medication.

Expel air from the syringe.

To ensure correct volume and to avoid
the introduction of air into the vein.

N.B. Medication must not be sprayed
into the atmosphere.

To prevent development of resistent
strains of micro-organisms.

Take the prescription sheet, swab and
loaded syringes in a receiver to the
patient.

To maintain safety.

Check the identity of the patient
against the prescription sheet (see
Oral Drug Administration procedure
(Chapter 36) and Health Authority
policy).

To maintain safety.

Position patient appropriately.

To allow easy access to cannula.

Recheck site of cannula prior to the
administration of the drug.

Prior to administration, cleanse the entry port with an alcohol-based swab.	To remove debris and to reduce the risk of infection.
Flush cannula with 1 ml sodium chloride 0.9 per cent.	To ensure patency. If not patent, inform medical staff.
Administer prescribed drug. N.B. Always adhere to manufacturer's instructions regarding the speed of administration.	
Reflush cannula using 1 ml sodium chloride 0.9 per cent.	To clear cannula.
Accountable nurse signs the prescription sheet.	To record drug administration.

Evaluation

Potential problems of procedure	**Appropriate nursing action**
Localised reaction to the drug, e.g. pain or burning sensation.	Stop giving the drug.
	Allay patient anxiety.
	Discontinue procedure and inform medical staff.
Adverse reaction to the drug.	This may be immediate – seek medical advice.
	Be prepared for resuscitation.
Blocked cannula.	Inform medical staff.

Adaptations for home care

This procedure is not applicable to the community.

References and further reading

British Intravenous Therapy Association (1986), *Guidelines for the Preparation of Nurses for Intravenous Drug Administration and Associated Intravenous Therapy*, Travenol Laboratories, Baxter Health Care Ltd, Caxton Way, Thetford, Norfolk, IP24 3SE.
Hecker, J. (1988), 'Improved technique in I.V. therapy', *Nursing Times*, vol. 84, no. 34, pp. 28–33.

28 Intravenous infusion

Definition

The administration of fluid and electrolytes directly into a vein. N.B. This is a sterile procedure.

Assessment

Action	Rationale
Determine if the patient is right- or left-handed.	To enable full use of dominant arm.
Determine if the area surrounding site of infusion is excessively hairy and requires clipping with scissors.	To reduce discomfort when the tape securing the cannula is removed.
Determine the need for more suitable night attire prior to commencement of the procedure.	To facilitate washing and dressing after the commencement of the infusion.
Determine if any additives are to be given via the infusion.	The use of an end line intravenous filter is recommended to prevent the risk of contamination.

Planning

Equipment

Prescribed solution for infusion.
Appropriate intravenous cannula.
Disposable intravenous giving set.
Alcohol-impregnated swab.
Tourniquet/sphygmomanometer.

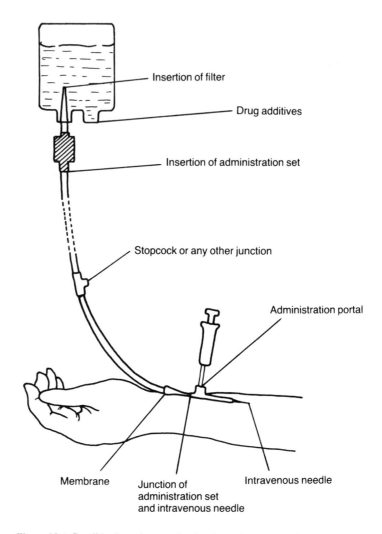

Figure 28.1 Possible sites of contamination for an intravenous infusion.

Adhesive tape.
Intravenous infusion stand.
Crepe bandage ⎱ only necessary if the cannula is sited near to the bend of
Splint ⎰ the elbow or the patient is very restless.
Fluid balance chart.
Disposal bag.
Local anaesthetic.
2 ml syringe and needle.
Scissors.

Implementation

Action	Rationale
Explain the procedure to the patient.	To obtain consent and co-operation and reduce anxiety.
Remove the outer covering and check that the intravenous solution prescribed is: • Within the expiry date. • Not cloudy. • Free of debris. • Undamaged.	To avoid misadministration and reduce the risk of adverse reaction to the infused solution, and avoid administering contaminated fluid.
Remove the protective outlet covering and suspend container from the intravenous infusion stand.	For ease of access.
Close the clamp on the giving set.	To control the movement of fluid.
Insert the cannula of the giving set into the bag of solution via the entry portal, ensuring asepsis.	To facilitate procedure.
Prime the giving set by squeezing and releasing the filter chamber until the lower chamber is half full.	To minimise air bubbles collecting in the system.
Flush tubing with fluid by slowly opening and closing the clamp.	To reduce the risk of air bubbles.
Assist doctor as required to connect and secure system to the intravenous cannula ensuring asepsis.	
Transiderm patch could be applied over cannulated vein.	To ensure vasodilation and prevent spasm and subsequent blockage.
Regulate flow of fluid as prescribed (see calculation formula shown below).	

Calculation formula

$$\frac{\text{Total volume of the prescribed fluid in ml}}{\text{Prescribed number of hours infusion is to take}} \times \frac{\text{Number of drops per ml}}{60} \text{(see information on giving set)} = \frac{\text{Number of drops}}{\text{to be infused/min}}$$

e.g. $\dfrac{1000}{8} \times \dfrac{20}{60} = 41$ drops/min

Record on appropriate chart type and quantity of fluid and time commenced.	To maintain an accurate record and assist in monitoring fluid balance.
Dispose of all equipment according to Health Authority policy.	To prevent injury to staff.

Evaluation

Potential problems of procedure	Indications	Appropriate nursing action
Extravasation of the cannula.	Pain and swelling at entry point and possibly a decrease in the flow rate.	Stop the infusion and inform medical staff. Elevate the arm to promote venous drainage and reduce oedema.
Phlebitis (inflammation of the vein).	Pain, a local increase in skin temperature and redness along the path of vein.	Stop infusion and inform the medical staff.
Slow or absent flow rate.	No obvious localised signs.	Expose the cannula and inspect the entry site for signs of inflammation and leakage. Examine the giving set for kinking. Reposition the arm.

N.B. If the above measures are unsuccessful inform the medical staff. Squeezing or flushing fluid through the cannula can be dangerous and cause extreme discomfort to the patient.

Blood in the giving set.	Elevate the arm on a pillow to prevent back flow.
Impaired circulation due to arm splinted in an unnatural position.	Remove splint at regular intervals to give passive physiotherapy to arm.
Administration of intravenous fluids in excess of 48 hours.	Giving set should be changed every 48 hours and cannula resited every 72 hours.

Adaptations for home care

This procedure is not applicable in the community.

References and further reading

Clutton-Brock, T.H. (1984), 'How to set up a drip and keep it going', *British Journal of Hospital Medicine*, vol. 32(4), pp. 162–7.

Francombe, P. (1988), 'Intravenous filters and phlebitis', *Nursing Times*, vol. 84(26), pp. 34–5.

Hecker, J. (1988), 'Improved technique in intra venous therapy', *Nursing Times*, vol. 84(34), pp. 28–33.

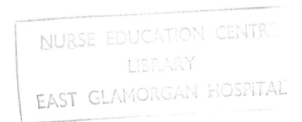

29   Last offices

Definition

The immediate care given to a patient when death has been confirmed by the medical staff.

Aim

To care for the body in a sensitive way, by cleansing and labelling in preparation for transfer to the Chapel of Rest or mortuary.

Assessment

Question	Action	Rationale
Who needs to be informed of the death?	Inform medical and senior nursing staff.	To certify death.
		For support and guidance and to ensure accurate records.
What are the wishes of the relatives?	Contact next of kin, if they are not present.	To ensure all relevant family members and friends are informed.
	Discuss the wishes of the family if not previously known.	To ensure that the wishes of the relatives are carried out.
		To assist in the bereavement process.

Are there any cultural or religious observances that need to be taken into account?	Check with relatives/ religious adviser/ relevant handbooks.	To avoid unnecessary offence or distress.
Is the body infectious?	Observe Health Authority policy re cadaver bags.	To reduce risk of cross-infection.
Was this death expected?	The medical staff will make appropriate decisions regarding the coroner or post mortem examination.	To meet legal obligations and confirm cause of death.
Are there any orifices/ wounds likely to discharge/drainage tubes/intravenous lines?	Seek and follow medical staff advice.	To prevent leakage and meet legal requirements.

Planning

Action	**Rationale**
Ensure privacy.	To maintain dignity of deceased and minimise distress to other patients.
Collect equipment to wash/shave/ groom body (refer to Bathing procedure in Chapter 6).	To ensure that relatives have as pleasant a memory as possible.
Collect shroud and clean sheets, observing cultural and family requirements.	To dress and cover body.
Collect appropriate documentation to label body and personal effects.	To ensure correct identification of body.
	To minimise possible loss of property and ensure correct 'handing over' to relatives.

Implementation

Action	Rationale
Contact relatives and friends and inform of death.	Quick contact minimises distress.
Straighten body, lie flat with one pillow under head.	To prevent collection of fluid in face, causing distortion.
Support jaw with small pillow on chest.	To prevent jaw sagging.
Close eyes (cover temporarily with wet cotton wool if eyes will not stay closed). Replace dentures if appropriate.	To maintain natural appearance of face.
Cover wounds as instructed.	To keep body clean (see Assessment section in this chapter).
Wash body as necessary. Dress in shroud. Change bed linen as necessary.	For aesthetic reasons.
Handle body carefully.	To prevent bruising.
List property in relevant documents with a witness and keep securely.	A record can be checked later if there is any discrepancy as theft can easily occur in hospital.
Deal with all valuables, including wedding ring, according to Health Authority policy.	To prevent unnecessary loss or misunderstanding.
Complete nursing records before the body is removed from the ward or department.	To ensure accurate records.
Take account of feelings of other patients/relatives when body is removed from the ward.	
Explain what has happened if appropriate.	Hiding facts can cause unnecessary anxiety.

Allow other patients to express their grief, anxiety and fears.

Evaluation

Potential problems of procedure

Relatives' distress.

Appropriate nursing action

The care for the patient is very often evaluated through the relatives. Regardless of whether the death was expected or not, the relatives will be experiencing their own bereavement process. It is important that they receive the correct information regarding property, death certificate and advice as to how to register the death and arrange a funeral.

This information is best received whilst they are sitting down and in private. A senior member of the nursing and medical staff needs to give time to do this possibly with refreshments. The spiritual needs of the bereaved should be considered at this time and the appropriate personnel involved.

Although a cup of tea is a British social conformity, it also gives focus for concentration and helps counteract the shock factor. Help received at this time is known to minimise trauma and aid a smoother passage through the bereavement process. Time is needed for the relatives to talk and to absorb the shock as they feel the need. Skill is required by the person with them at this time to counsel and to give 'space', silence, verbal and/or non-verbal support.

Staff distress.

Staff should be given the opportunity to express their own feelings with appropriate support.

Adaptations for home care

This procedure is unlikely in the community.

References and further reading

Ayrton, N.A. (1982), 'Last offices in cases of notifiable disease', *The Journal of Infection Control Nursing, Nursing Times*, 12 May, pp. 5–6.

Ball, M. (1976), *Death*, Oxford University Press in association with Chameleon/Ikon, Oxford.

Bell, I. (1984), 'Bereavement in continuing care wards', *Nursing Times*, 12 September, pp. 51–2.

Conboy-Hill, S. (1986), 'Terminal care – their death in your hands', *The Professional Nurse*, November, pp. 51–3.

McGuiness, S. (1986), 'Death rites', *Nursing Times*, 19 March, pp. 28–31.

Pennington, E. (1978), 'Post mortem care – more than a ritual', *American Journal of Nursing*, May, pp. 846–7.

Religions and Cultures – A Guide to Patients' Beliefs and Customs for Health Service Staff, (1984), revised edn, Lothian Community Relations Council, Edinburgh.

Storr, E. (1986), 'Practical details the survivors have to face', *Geriatric Medicine*, June, pp. 40–4.

What to do After Death, Leaflet D49, Department of Health and Social Security.

30 Lifting

Definition

To move a patient with minimal effort avoiding injury to both patient and staff. There is less risk of injury to the patient, colleagues and the nurse when flat well-supported shoes are worn, clothing is loose, jewellery and wrist watches are not worn and nails are short. Please refer to the Health Authority uniform policy.

Assessment

Action	Rationale
Determine the reason for procedure.	To ensure correct lift is selected. (See Figure 30.1)
Assess whether additional personnel/ equipment will be needed dependent upon the patient's weight, condition and ability.	To facilitate easy movement and to avoid injury to patient and staff.
Determine how much the patient can do to assist in the procedure.	To facilitate independence.
Make sure bed space is clear of obstacles and the floor is not wet.	To prevent accidents.

N.B. It is not recommended to use an orthodox lift, as this puts too much strain on the nurse's back. Two nurses lifting the patient's trunk and two nurses lifting the pelvis and legs is recommended as an alternative.

Common lifts	Indications for use	Contraindications
Shoulder or Australian lift (Figure 30.3)	Lift of choice; may need to be adapted for hemiplegic patients.	Damage to patient's upper trunk. Inability to sit forward or co-operate.
Three-person lift (Figure 30.4)	Used to transfer patients from bed to bed, or bed to trolley; useful for patients who cannot sit up.	Insufficient staff for the weight of the patient.
Pivot transfer (Figure 30.5); this should only be used following an assessment by a physiotherapist.	Patients following a stroke, who have some ability to stand/balance. Can be used with one nurse.	Patient's inability to co-operate. When patient much taller than the nurse. Leg spasms.
Through-arm lift (Figure 30.6)	Patient with extensive paralysis/neuropathies.	Chest injuries or surgery. Flaccid shoulders, painful shoulders with no active movement.

Figure 30.1 Chart to be used in assessment.

Planning

Action	**Rationale**
Ensure that the correct number of personnel of a similar height are available.	To avoid injury to staff and patients.

Equipment

Select the suitable equipment according to the assessment, e.g. ambulift, hoist, 'monkey pole'.

Check and/or adjust equipment to ensure optimum safety and comfort.

Implementation

General principles of lifting

Action	**Rationale**
Explain the procedure to the patient.	To gain co-operation and alleviate anxiety.
Encourage the patient to help where	To avoid strain and injury and to

appropriate.	facilitate independence.
Position relevant equipment close to the patient allowing room for manoeuvre.	To minimise effort and maximise safety.
Ensure the wheels on any equipment are locked.	To avoid accidents.
Ensure that the bed is adjusted to a height suitable for both lifters.	To minimise effort and maximise safety.
Select one person to lead and give instructions.	To avoid confusion and to ensure everyone lifts in unison.
Stand with feet apart.	To maintain balance.
Bend knees, keeping back straight and vertical.	To avoid back injury.
Avoid twisting or bending from the waist.	To minimise strain on the back and abdominal muscles.
Ensure patient is held in close proximity.	To maintain balance and facilitate lift.
Maintain a firm grasp but not too tight (see Figure 30.2).	To avoid undue pressure to lifting partner.
Avoid dragging or pinching the patient's skin.	To avoid damage to the skin.

Shoulder lift or Australian lift (Figure 30.3)

Action	Rationale
Position the patient leaning forward, with knees slightly flexed.	To allow easy access for the nurse.
Position two nurses, one on each side of the bed.	To facilitate procedure.
Each nurse should stand:	To avoid injury
• Close to bed.	
• At level of the patient's hips.	

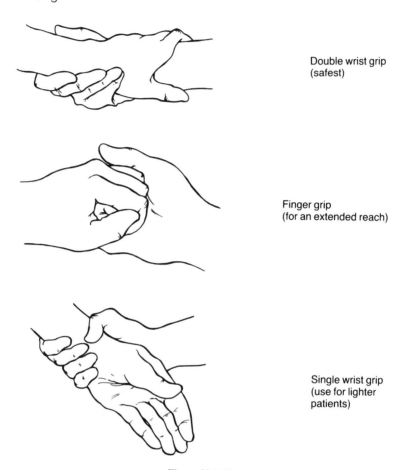

Double wrist grip
(safest)

Finger grip
(for an extended reach)

Single wrist grip
(use for lighter
patients)

Figure 30.2 Suggested grasps.

- Facing the head of the bed.
- With feet apart.
- With leading foot facing in the
  direction of the lift.

Each nurse should: To facilitate lift and avoid injury.

- Bend their knees.
- Place the arm nearest to the
  patient high under the patient's
  thighs.
- Grasp partner's wrist securely.
- Press the shoulder into the

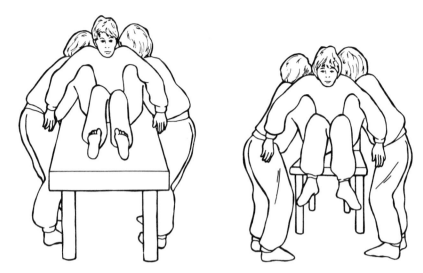

Figure 30.3 Shoulder lift or Australian lift.

patient's axilla.
- Place free hand on mattress or bed head.
- Straightening knees or hips, transfer weight to forward leg.
- Lift patient clear of the bed.

N.B. The patient's co-operation by placing their arms down the nurses' backs is essential.

Lifting the patient from bed to chair (Figure 30.3)

Action	Rationale
Lift the patient to the side of the bed.	To facilitate procedure.
The nurse nearest to the chair supports the patient. The second nurse repositions by the patient (proceed to lift as described above).	To facilitate procedure.

This lift may be used for a patient with a hemiplegia, where the affected arm is kept to their side and the nurse presses close to the body.

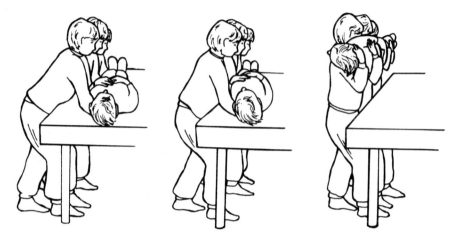

Figure 30.4 Three-person lift.

Three-person lift (Figure 30.4)

Action	Rationale
An unoccupied trolley or bed is positioned with the head at the foot of the occupied bed.	For easy transfer.
Adjust the bed height to maximum and apply brakes.	To avoid injury to patient and nurse.
Position the three lifters on the same side of the bed as the unoccupied trolley, with strongest person in the middle.	For even distribution of weight.
The first lifter at the head cradles the head of the patient and supports the shoulders and upper back.	For even distribution of weight.
The second lifter in the middle supports lower back and buttocks.	For even distribution of weight.
The third lifter at the feet supports thighs and legs.	For even distribution of weight.

N.B. For a very heavy patient, more lifters may be needed.	To redistribute weight more evenly.
Lifters place their forearms gently under the patient.	To facilitate procedure.
When taking the weight of the patient, the lifters should place the same foot forward as close to the bed as possible and bend their knees.	To maintain balance.
Lifters transfer the weight by lifting in unison and cradle the patient against their chests.	To maximise a safe efficient lift.
The lifters move in unison towards the unoccupied trolley and, bending their knees, gently lower the patient on to the trolley.	To avoid confusion and maximise safety.

Pivot transfer (Figure 30.5)

Action

With the patient seated, rock the patient from side to side and pull alternate legs forward from the pelvis.

Rationale

To assist the patient to the front of the seat.

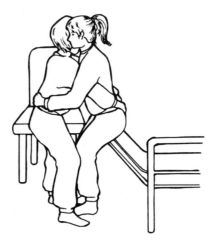

Figure 30.5 Pivot transfer.

Position the patient's feet on the floor at right angles to the knees.

To enable the weight to come forward over the base of the spine.

The nurse stands with feet in a V-shape blocking the patient's weak knee with their knee.

To prevent foot/feet slipping and to strengthen the weak knee(s).

N.B. If both patient's legs are weak, nurse must block both knees together.

Hold the patient as follows:

      Arm 1 – place under patient's good arm and around scapula.

To facilitate procedure.

      Arm 2 – place around patient's bottom as support.

To facilitate procedure.

N.B. Nurse must maintain lumbar lordosis.

To avoid injury.

Bring patient forward into standing position and move the hemiplegic side forward into the chair.

N.B. Patient may be moved good side forward depending on disability (check with physiotherapist).

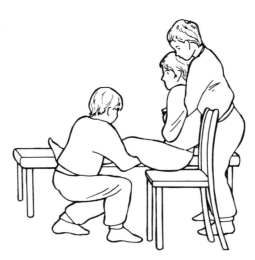

Figure 30.6 Through-arm lift (see Figure 30.1).

Evaluation

Potential problems of procedure	Appropriate nursing action
Injury to staff and patients.	Choose the correct lift for the size and condition of the patient and ensure sufficient lifters.
Actual injury occurring.	Immediately inform line manager and document appropriately (according to Health Authority policy).
	Seek medical advice.
	If injury to staff, inform union representative.
Cot sides *in situ*.	Remove or retract prior to procedure.
Insufficient staff to maintain safe lifting practice.	Inform nurse manager. Never attempt to lift unassisted.

Adaptations for home care

Ensure correct equipment is available, e.g. hoist or monkey pole. Explain to carer the reasons for lifting the patient. Teach them to help and how to lift and make patients comfortable between district nurse visits.

1. *The Australian lift* – the lift should not be attempted unless there are two nurses or the carer has been taught and is able to fully co-operate.
2. *Three-person lift* – this lift is not carried out in the community.
3. *Pivot transfer* – carried out as procedure.

References and further reading

Lifting and Moving Patients Safely, (1986), Scriptographic Publications Ltd, Haslemere, Surrey.
Troup, J.D.G. *et al.* (1988), *The Handling of Patients, a Guide for Nurses*, 2nd edn, National Back Pain Association, in association with the Royal College of Nursing, London.

31   Lumbar puncture

Definition

Insertion of a needle into the lumbar subarachnoid space for the purpose of withdrawing cerebro-spinal fluid for diagnostic or therapeutic reasons.

Assessment

Action	Rationale
Assess condition of patient, i.e. conscious/unconscious.	To facilitate adequate psychological preparation and explanation of procedure.
Determine reason for procedure.	To facilitate adequate preparation of patient and equipment.

Planning

Equipment

> On a trolley, as for a sterile procedure.
> Lumbar puncture pack.
> Lumbar puncture needle.
> 5 ml syringe and needles.
> Local anaesthetic.
> Skin tincture, e.g. chlorhexidine 0.5 per cent.
> Skin sealant.
> Waterproof plaster.
> Sterile gloves (one pair).
> Three universal containers and laboratory forms.
> Disposal bag.

Action	**Rationale**
Explain procedure to patient.	To obtain co-operation and consent.
	Restless patients and children may need sedation.
Prepare trolley maintaining aseptic technique.	To facilitate procedure and maintain sterility throughout.

Implementation

Action	**Rationale**
Place patient in the optimum position maintaining comfort, warmth and privacy.	To facilitate easy access to lumbar spine and widen intervertebral spaces.
Usually flat, one pillow. Firm mattress. Lateral to edge of bed. Head and neck flexed. Knees drawn up to chest. Lumbar area exposed.	To facilitate easy access to lumbar spine and widen intervertebral spaces.
Comfort, support and observe patient throughout procedure.	To maintain patient co-operation and position. Sudden movement may produce blood stained specimen.
Assist doctor as required with:	
• Recording cerebro-spinal fluid pressure readings.	To determine any deviation from the normal. Normal pressure is $60-180$ mm H_2O.
• Compression of jugular veins. Queckenstedt's manoeuvre.	To check for obstruction to cerebro-spinal fluid in spinal column.
• Obtaining appropriate specimens of cerebro-spinal fluid. Checking they are correctly labelled and sent to the laboratory immediately.	To facilitate early diagnosis.
Apply small adhesive plaster to puncture site.	To protect the patient's night-clothes and to minimise the risk of infection.
Reposition patient after procedure.	To facilitate patient's comfort.

Evaluation

Potential problems of procedure	Appropriate nursing action
Herniation (coning).	Observe vital and neurological signs.
Headache due to loss of cerebro-spinal fluid.	Give analgesia as prescribed and increase fluid intake.
Infection.	Observe temperature during subsequent 24 hours.
Leakage of cerebro-spinal fluid from puncture site.	Report to medical staff immediately.

Adaptations for home care

This procedure is not applicable in the community.

References and further reading

Jamieson, E., McCall, J. and Blythe, R. (1988), *Guidelines for Clinical Nursing Practices*, Churchill Livingstone, Edinburgh, pp. 66–71.
Pritchard, A.P. and Walker, V.A. (eds.) *The Royal Marsden Hospital Manual of Clinical Nursing Policies and Procedures*, (1984), Harper & Row, London, pp. 268–272.

32   Naso-gastric intubation and aspiration

Definition

The passing of a tube via the nose into the stomach.

Assessment

Action	Rationale

Determine the reason for the procedure:

- Prior to or following abdominal surgery.

  To ensure stomach is empty and to relieve the anastomosis of pressure.

- Persistent vomiting.

  To reduce the risk of aspiration and facilitate patient comfort.

- Intestinal obstruction.

  To empty stomach of contents and facilitate patient comfort.

Planning

Equipment

Naso-gastric tube, e.g. Ryle's tube, sizes 12, 14, 16 F.G.
Lubrication.
Blue litmus paper.
Receiver.
50 ml syringe (with catheter mount tip).
Adhesive tape.
Drainage bag.
Spigot.
Disposal bag.
Tissues.

Action	Rationale
Explain reason and nature of the procedure to the patient.	To gain consent and co-operation and reduce anxiety.

Implementation

Action	Rationale
Ensure privacy.	To reduce anxiety and embarrassment.
Select the most appropriate position, usually upright.	To facilitate passing the tube.
Ensure the nostrils are clean.	To facilitate passing the tube.
Measure the tube to determine the length necessary to allow entry to the stomach. Nose to xiphisternum.	To ensure correct position of tube and to facilitate drainage.
Lubricate the tube and encourage the patient to swallow when requested.	To enable easy passage of the tube.
Pass the tube gently into stomach via the nose.	To reduce the risk of naso-oesophageal trauma.
Aspirate with a syringe and test contents with blue litmus paper.	To ensure the tube is in the stomach (the litmus paper should turn pink).
Secure the tube to the patient's nose and cheek with a small piece of adhesive tape.	To ensure the tube does not move and to maximise comfort and cosmetic effect.
Aspirate the tube using a syringe until no further aspirate can be obtained.	
Attach drainage bag or spigot to the tube.	To allow continuous drainage from the stomach or to prevent leakage, respectively.
Ensure drainage bag is below level of stomach.	To facilitate drainage by siphonage.

Record the volume and nature of the aspirate on the appropriate documentation.

To ensure accurate monitoring of fluid balance.

Evaluation

Potential problems of procedure

Appropriate nursing action

No aspirate.

Ensure correct positioning of the tube by:

- Checking the back of the throat for coiling.
- Diverting the end of the tube under water.

N.B. Air bubbles corresponding with respiration indicates the tube is in the lungs.

Reposition the patient in the left lateral position and reaspirate.

Tube misplaced outside the stomach.

Remove and recommence procedure, if the patient's condition allows.

Sore throat.

Give ice chips or mouth washes as patient's condition allows.

Adaptations for home care

This procedure is not applicable in the community.

References and further reading

Jamieson, E., McCall, J. and Blythe, R. (1988), *Guidelines for Clinical Nursing Practices*, Churchill Livingstone, Edinburgh.
Volden, C., Grinde, J. and Carl, D. (1980), 'Taking the trauma out of nasogastric intubation', *Nursing*, vol. 10(9), pp. 14–17.

33 Naso-pharyngeal/oro-pharyngeal suction

Definition

Removal of respiratory tract secretions from naso-oropharynx for a patient who is unable to expectorate efficiently.

Assessment

Action	Rationale
Assess respiratory function for:	To establish the need for suction.
• Rate, rhythm, cyanosis. • Presence of audible rhonchi. • Inability to expectorate independently.	N.B. Only apply suction when absolutely necessary, to prevent complications.
N.B. Liaise with physiotherapist where appropriate.	
Assess appropriate size of suction catheter necessary, e.g. size 12 F.G. for adult use.	To minimise risk of trauma.

Planning

Equipment

Suction apparatus, tubing and 'Y' connector.
Sterile suction catheters.
Sterile disposable gloves.
Single use gallipot with sterile water for flushing.
Tissues.
Disposal bag.

Action	Rationale
Test suction pressure by kinking the suction tubing and alter gauge appropriately.	To minimise risk of trauma and hypoxia.

Naso-pharyngeal

Adults 120–150 mm Hg.
Infants/small children 60–100 mm Hg.
Older children 100–120 mm Hg.

Oro-pharyngeal

Adults – pressures up to 300 mm Hg.
Children – pressures up to 200 mm Hg.

Action	Rationale
Explain procedure to the patient and ensure privacy.	To allay fears and gain co-operation.
Position patient appropriately (either upright if conscious or laterally if unconscious).	To facilitate aspiration of secretions.

Implementation

Action	Rationale
Connect suction catheter to suction apparatus, leaving catheter in sterile packet.	To maintain sterility.
Glove dominant hand, remove catheter from packet and handle with gloved hand.	To maintain sterility.
Lubricate catheter tip with sterile water soluble gel if using nasal approach.	To reduce resistance to catheter entry. To minimise trauma to nasal mucosa.
With 'Y' connector open, pass suction catheter into nose or mouth for approximately 3–4 in. (7.5–10 cm) oro-pharyngeal; 5–6 in. (12.5–15 cm) naso-pharyngeal.	To prevent suction on insertion of catheter.

N.B. In the absence of a 'Y' connection, kink tubing during insertion of catheter.

If using nasal approach, and resistance is met try other nostril. Do not use force.	To prevent trauma.
Cover 'Y' connector, rotate and gently withdraw suction catheter.	To facilitate efficient suction and passage of catheter.
Apply suction for a maximum of 15 seconds only.	To prevent hypoxia occurring.

N.B. Suction should only be applied when withdrawing catheter.

Flush catheter with sterile water.	To prevent blockage of equipment.
Allow patient time to breathe deeply.	To prevent hypoxia occurring.
Repeat suction procedure if necessary.	To fully clear the airway.
Invert glove over catheter and discard into disposal bag.	To prevent cross-infection.

Evaluation

Potential problems of procedure	**Appropriate nursing action**
Fresh blood on suction/coughing.	Inform medical staff. Administer oxygen if prescribed. Apply gentle suction as necessary to maintain airway.
Sudden deterioration in patient's condition, e.g. cyanosis, air hunger, restlessness.	Stop suction.
	Inform medical staff.
	Administer oxygen.
	Check vital signs and record.

Adaptations for home care

Procedure is carried out as described above.

References and further reading

Allen, D. (1988), 'Making sense of suctioning', *Nursing Times*, vol. 84(10), pp. 46–7.

Birdsall, C. (1985), 'What suction pressure should I use?', *American Journal of Nursing*, vol. 5, p. 866.

Hoffman, L.A. *et al.* (1988), 'Airway management for the critically ill patient', *American Journal of Nursing*, vol. 1, pp. 39–53.

34   Nebulisation

Definition

Reducing a liquid to a fine spray using compressed air or oxygen.

Aims

1. To moisten secretions in the respiratory tract.
2. To facilitate expectoration or suction.
3. To administer drugs.

Assessment

Action	Rationale
Determine reason for procedure.	To enable relevant equipment to be assembled.

Planning

Equipment

Air cylinder, compressed air generator or oxygen.
Appropriate mask.
Tubing.
Tissues.
For moistening secretions – nebuliser, sterile distilled water.
To administer drug – mini-nebuliser, appropriate drug (see Oral Drug
Administration procedure, Chapter 36).

Action	Rationale
Explain the procedure to the patient.	To gain consent and co-operation and reduce anxiety.
N.B. The procedure can be very noisy.	
Assemble relevant equipment.	To facilitate procedure.

Implementation

Action	Rationale
Place mask in the appropriate position.	To ensure airway is covered.
Set oxygen/air to prescribed rate.	To ensure nebulisation occurs.

Evaluation

Potential problems of procedure	Appropriate nursing action
Chafing of face.	Relieve pressure by loosening padding/mask.
Claustrophobia.	Give patient a detailed description of procedure and length of time necessary.
Excessive moisture in respiratory tract.	Discontinue treatment and seek appropriate nursing/medical advice.
Infection. N.B. The nebuliser is a potential source of gram negative organisms.	Use disposable nebuliser or equipment which can be sterilised. Always empty, clean and dry equipment between use throughout the day.

The effectiveness of treatment should always be noted in the patient's records.

Adaptations for home care

This procedure may be conducted in the community as outlined above. Relatives and patient should be taught regarding the safe use and storage of equipment and the correct methods of obtaining supplies and disposing of equipment.

Reference and further reading

Jamieson, E., McCall, J. and Blythe, R. (1988), *Guidelines for Clinical Nursing Practices*, Churchill Livingstone, Edinburgh.

35 Neurological observations

Definition

An assessment of the patient's conscious level and nervous system co-ordination.

Aim

To monitor and evaluate the patient's condition by observing a combination of the following:

Level of consciousness.
Vital signs of blood pressure, pulse, temperature and respiration.
Pupillary activity.
Motor function.
Sensory function.

Assessment

Action	Rationale
Assess the condition of the patient.	To facilitate appropriate explanation of the procedure at any conscious level.
Determine reasons for observations in order to determine frequency of observation and identify appropriate observation.	To monitor the patient's condition and prevent undue disturbance.

Planning

Equipment

Pen torch.
Sphygmomanometer.
Thermometer/probe.
Appropriate chart.

Implementation – Utilising the Glasgow Coma Scale

Action	Rationale
Explain the observation to the patient.	The sense of hearing may be unimpaired even when the patient is unconscious.
	To ensure the patient as far as possible understands and consents to the observation.
Ask the patient to open their eyes.	To monitor the response of the patient to the spoken voice and to determine the patient's physical ability to open their eyes.
Assess the pupil responses.	To evaluate size, shape, equality and reaction to light (see Evaluation).
Ask the patient the day, year and place.	To assess the patient's level of orientation.
Ask the patient to carry out a simple command.	To determine the patient's ability to carry out verbal commands.
Take the patient's blood pressure and pulse.	To monitor and detect signs of raised intracranial pressure (see Evaluation).
Ask the patient to grasp and release your hand. Ask the patient to lift their leg off the bed.	To assess degree and equality of motor function.
Record observations on the appropriate chart.	For early detection of abnormalities and to enable appropriate intervention.

Report any changes to nurse in charge.   To enable appropriate intervention.

Evaluation

Potential problems of the procedure	Rationale	Appropriate nursing action
Conscious level deteriorating.	Impaired brain functioning due to trauma or pressure.	Inform nurse in charge and medical officer.
Raised blood pressure.	Intracranial pressure rising.	Inform nurse in charge and medical officer.
Slowing pulse.	Intracranial pressure rising.	Inform nurse in charge and medical officer.
Unequal pupils.	Eye injury or an enlarging intracranial swelling or mass causing pressure on optic nerve.	Inform nurse in charge and medical officer.
Slow reaction of pupils to light.	Intracranial pressure on ocular motor nerve.	Inform nurse in charge and medical officer.
Dilating pupil/pupils.	Enlarging intracranial mass or swelling causing gradual occlusion of ocular motor nerve.	Inform nurse in charge and medical officer.
Limb/limbs not responding to commands/painful stimuli.	Damage/pressure to corresponding section of brain/spinal cord.	Inform nurse in charge and medical officer.
Rise in temperature.	Interference or trauma to the heat regulating centre.	Inform nurse in charge and medical officer.
Change in rate, rhythm and ratio of inspiration/expiration.	Severe intracranial pressure.	Inform nurse in charge and medical officer.

Adaptations for home care

This procedure is unlikely to be conducted in the community.

References and further reading

Jones, C. (1979), 'Glasgow coma scale', *American Journal of Nursing*, vol. 79(9), pp. 1551–3.

Ladyshewsky, A. (1980), 'Increased intracranial pressure – when assessment counts', *The Canadian Nurse*, vol. 76(9), pp. 34–7.

Teasdale, G. (1975), 'Acute impairment of brain functions 1: assessing conscious level', *Nursing Times*, vol. 71(24), pp. 914–17.

Teasdale, G., Galbraith, S. and Clarke, K. (1975), 'Acute impairment of brain functions 2: observation record chart', *Nursing Times*, vol. 71(25), pp. 972–3.

36   Oral drug administration

Definition

The safe and correct giving of prescribed drugs via the mouth to a patient by an accountable nurse. Types of drugs given orally are:

1. Capsule – medication given in powder form surrounded by soluble case usually made of gelatin.
2. Tablet – medication given in a compressed form.
3. Lozenge – medication given in a dissolvable sugar base, usually sucked slowly by the patient to allow medication to be applied to mouth and throat.
4. Elixir – medication given in a liquid form, usually to facilitate administration to patients with swallowing difficulties.
5. Granules – medication given in small grain-like particles.
6. Sublingual – medication in tablet form given under the tongue for speedy absorption.

N.B. This procedure must be used in conjunction with the Health Authority policy for the prescribing, handling, custody and administration of drugs.

Assessment

Action	Rationale
Assess the condition of the patient.	To ensure that the patient is able to take their medication orally.
	To aid evaluation after the drug has been given.
Assess patient's knowledge of the drug being given.	To facilitate appropriate explanation. A patient should know any potential effects of the drug.

Determine category of drug to be given, e.g. controlled drug.	To determine legal requirements and Health Authority policy.

N.B. Sugar coated drugs for delayed absorption must not be crushed or chewed.

Planning

Equipment

> Medicine trolley and appropriate keys.
> Calibrated medicine containers.
> Jug of water and tumblers.
> Disposal bag.
> Bowl of soapy water.
> Drug formulary.
> Spoons.

Action	**Rationale**
Select opimum position for patient, preferably sitting up.	To facilitate administration of drug.

Implementation

Action	**Rationale**
The procedure should always involve a nurse who is qualified and/or deemed an accountable person according to Health Authority policy.	To meet legal requirements and Health Authority policy.
Read the prescription. Ascertain which drug is due to be given.	To determine whether one or two nurses are required to check the drug (see Health Authority policy).
Check that the prescription is correctly and legibly written and signed by medical staff.	To minimise the risk of error and to protect the patient.
Select the drug required and check expiry date.	Drugs may no longer be effective after the expiry date.

If the drug is labelled 'Controlled Drug', check that the number of tablets/ampoules corresponds with the balance in the controlled drug register.	To meet legal requirements and Health Authority policy.
Report any discrepancies immediately.	
Calculate the required dosage.	
Place the required dose into the container, avoiding contact with hands.	To prevent cross-infection.
Check the patient's identity, using identity band for name and registration number which must correspond with the prescription sheet.	To prevent misadministration of drug.
Explain to patient: • What drug is being given. • Route of administration. • Any possible effects.	To ensure the patient has full knowledge about their treatment. To obtain consent and co-operation.
Ascertain any specific instructions for giving the drug.	Some drugs may need to be given with milk or food to prevent gastric irritation.
Administer drugs to be swallowed with a drink of water.	To facilitate swallowing and reduce the risk of oesophageal damage.
Sign the prescription chart according to Health Authority policy.	To meet legal requirements and Health Authority policy. To provide an accurate record that the drug has been given.
Place the used container in the bowl of water. Ensure containers are washed and dried after use.	
Ensure medicine trolley is locked in place after use.	To meet legal requirements.

Evaluation

Action

Observe patient for any changes in condition and report to medical staff.

Rationale

To detect early complications due to drug interaction, sensitivity or toxicity.

To evaluate the effectiveness of the drug given.

Potential problems of procedure

Illegible prescription.

Identity band missing.

Patient absent from ward when drug is due.

Refusal of drug.

Unconscious patient with naso-gastric tube.

Day patients.

Appropriate nursing action

Refer to nursing and medical staff and withhold administration of the drug.

Refer to medical notes. Check name, address and date of birth and write new name band, taking registration number from the medical notes. Place identity band on patient's wrist. Continue with procedure.

Inform nurse in charge. Record non-administration on prescription sheet. Check with nurse in charge regarding administration of drug on patient's return.

Ascertain reason for refusal.

Record non-administration.

Inform medical staff.

Dispose of drug according to Health Authority policy.

Refer to enteral feeding procedure.

All drugs given to the patient should be clearly prescribed by the doctor on the patient's prescription sheet.

Refer to Health Authority policy.

Adaptations for home care

This procedure is not applicable in the community.

References and further reading

Adamson, L. (1978), 'Control of medicines in the U.K.', *Nursing Times*, vol. 74, pp. 973–5.

Bayliss, P.F.C. (1980), *Law on Poisons, Medicines and Related Substances*, 3rd edn, Ravenswood Publications, Beckenham, Kent.

Hopkins, S.J. (1983), *Drugs and Pharmacology for Nurses*, 8th edn, Churchill Livingstone, Edinburgh.

Recommended procedures for the normal prescribing, handling, custody and administration of drugs within the Central Birmingham Health Authority, 1986 Revision.

Thomas, S. (1979), 'Practical nursing – medicines: care and administration', *Nursing Mirror*, vol. 148(15), pp. 28–30.

37   Oral hygiene

Definition

The process of cleansing and freshening the mouth, teeth and gums.

Assessment

The amount of assistance required will be related to the state of dependency, age, limitations, mouth problems, etc., of the individual patient. The mouth needs to be inspected using a wooden spatula and a pen torch (an ordinary torch diffuses the light rays to give inadequate vision).

The following assessment guide provides a useful tool to assist with the planning of individualised patient care.

Treatments	Hydration state	Oral assessment	Dependency
	Hydrated	Mucous membrane, intact, healthy	Independent
	1	1	1
Drug therapy	Nil by mouth	Dentures Crusts/sordes present	Requires assistance
2	2	2	2
Oxygen therapy	Dehydrated	Dental caries Gum disease	Totally dependent
3	3	3	3

A score of four or above would indicate that special attention to the mouth is required.

Planning

Equipment

A Conscious, bedfast patient	B Unconscious patient	C The patient with dentures

Tooth-brush and paste
Receiver
Mouthwash/water
Paper towel
	Mouthwash solution
	Small head, soft
	  tooth-brush
	Pencil torch
	Disposable glove
	Gauze
	Foam sticks
	Paper towel
	Disposal bag
		Denture/tooth-brush
		Denture cleaner
		Denture container – with
		  the patient's name
		  on lid
		Bowl of cold water
		Mouthwash solution
		Receiver

Question	Action and rationale
Is the patient mouth breathing and/or dehydrated?	Give regular mouthwashes. Monitor fluid intake.
Does the patient have stomatitis, thrombocytopenia?	Use of a tooth-brush is contraindicated due to the risk of trauma.
Does the patient have sordes or crusts?	Use sodium bicarbonate solution. One teaspoon to 600 ml of warm water. This dissolves and loosens debris.
Does the patient have dry lips?	Apply yellow soft paraffin to lubricate lips.

Implementation

Action	Rationale
Consider the patient's preferences at all times.	This predisposes to individualised patient care and fosters the nurse–patient partnership.
Ensure privacy at all times.	To minimise patient's embarrassment.

The conscious, bedfast patient

Action	Rationale
Place the patient in a position that is appropriate to comfort and safety.	To facilitate the procedure and prevent the inhalation of the rinsing solution.
Assist the patient to brush the inside and outside of the teeth using the tooth-brush and paste. N.B. Teeth should be brushed four or five times in the direction of tooth growth in each part of the mouth.	To loosen debris, increase blood flow to the gums and minimise plaque formation.
Assist the patient to rinse the mouth with mouthwash solution or water, voiding the contents into the receiver. A straw may be used if necessary.	To remove loose debris and leave the mouth clean and fresh.
Document procedure in nursing records.	To assist with the evaluation of care.

The unconscious patient

Action	Rationale
Explain to the patient what you are about to do.	Although unconscious the patient may be able to hear and understand.
Turn the patient's head to the side.	To prevent inhalation of fluid.
Use normal saline to replace toothpaste.	To moisten the tooth-brush and avoid inhalation of toothpaste.
If the patient has their own teeth, these are gently brushed as for the conscious, bedfast patient.	To loosen debris, increase blood flow to the gums and minimise plaque formation.
N.B. Foam sticks can be used when a tooth-brush cannot be tolerated.	To promote patient's comfort and co-operation.
Using a gloved finger and a piece of gauze, clean cheek pouches.	To remove debris.
Using foam sticks, massage gums.	To stimulate the production of saliva.

The care of dentures

Action	Rationale
Assist the patient to remove the dentures. If patient unable to remove dentures, they should be removed by the nurse.	To release the suction holding the upper and lower plates in place.
The upper set can be removed by applying pressure with the tips of the index fingers to the top of the plate over the incisors.	To release the suction holding the upper and lower plates in place.
The lower set can be removed by applying slight pressure on the lower external edge of the plate. This is usually sufficient to release suction.	To release the suction holding the upper and lower plates in place.
Clean the dentures with a denture/ tooth-brush and cleanser/paste using an up and down movement.	To remove any debris thereby reducing the risk of oral infection and preventing the staining of the teeth.
Return the dentures, in a container of cold water, to the patient.	Moist dentures are easier to insert and are less likely to scratch the inside of the mouth.
Reinsert the dentures after giving the patient a mouthwash solution to rinse out the mouth.	To remove residual debris and prevent soreness and infection.
N.B. Reinsert dentures if possible.	If dentures are not worn for long periods of time, the gums will atrophy, resulting in ill-fitting dentures and problems with mastication.
Or store the clean dentures in fresh cold water, in a container labelled with patient's name.	To inhibit the multiplication of micro-organisms and prevent creaking and warping due to drying out of the plastic.
	To protect the patient's property from loss and damage.

Evaluation

Nursing actions must be recorded in the nursing records.

Potential problems of procedure	Appropriate nursing action
Crusts – Dried food and secretions.	See Planning section in this chapter.
Gingivitis – Inflammation of the gums.	Inform medical staff.
Glossitis – Inflammation of the tongue.	Inform medical staff.
Plaque – A mass of bacterial cells and other debris that adheres to the teeth.	Brush teeth regularly in the direction of tooth growth.
Sordes – Brown crusts which form on the lips of patients who consistently have a high temperature or who are dehydrated.	See Planning section in this chapter.
Stomatitis – Inflammation of the mouth.	Inform medical staff.
Halitosis – Bad breath.	Inform medical staff.
Parotitis – Inflammation of the salivary glands.	Inform medical staff.
Thrush – Infectious fungal infection of the mouth.	Inform medical staff.

Adaptations for home care

Patient and/or carers should be taught how to carry out this procedure correctly. Proprietary brands of mouthwash are available via retail chemists.

References and further reading

Dudjak, L.A. (1987), 'Mouth care for mucositis due to radiation therapy', *Cancer Nursing*, vol. 10(3), pp. 131–40.
Harrison, A. (1987), 'Denture care', *Nursing Times*, vol. 83(12), pp. 28–9.
Shepherd, G. *et al.* (1987), 'The mouth trap', *Nursing Times*, vol. 83(19), pp. 24–7.

38　　Oxygen therapy

Definition

The administration of oxygen through specialised equipment to increase tissue oxygenation. N.B. Oxygen is prescribed by a doctor who will decide the amount in litres and the percentage. Ideally, blood gases should be taken prior to use. Patients receiving oxygen should be in a position where they can be clearly observed by nursing staff and have call bell facilities.

Assessment

Action

Assess patient's condition.

Rationale

To ensure selection of most appropriate equipment.

Planning

Equipment

> Nasal cannulae or mask.
> Connection tubing.
> Flow meter.
> Oxygen supply, either piped or cylinder.
> Cylinders are black with white shoulders.
> Check there is an adequate supply of oxygen.
> NO SMOKING sign.
> Humidification may be needed.

N.B. Humidification of the oxygen supply to a venturi device (Ventimask) is not advised. Not only may this give inadequate humidification of the total inspired gas, but precipitation of water occurs within the venturi, thus altering the concentration delivered. Humidity adaptors are available from the manufacturers (see Table 38.1).

Table 38.1 Equipment available for oxygen therapy

Type	Description	Advantages
Nasal cannulae	A pair of tubes, 2 cm long. One fits into each nostril.	Less claustrophobic than a mask. Patient can eat, drink and speak normally.
Ventimask	A mask incorporating a device to enable a fixed concentration of oxygen to be delivered independent of patient factors or fit to the face. Oxygen is forced out through a small hole in the nozzle and comes out at high speed causing a venturi effect which enables air to mix with the oxygen.	When oxygen flow is set at the required rate, only the stated percentage will be given.
MC Mask	Mask has a soft plastic facepiece. Ventholes are provided to allow expired air to escape.	Used when high concentration of oxygen is needed but actual percentage not critical.
Humidifier	Various types available. Oxygen is moistened with sterile water before reaching the patient.	Prevents drying effect on mucous membranes.

Note: Different manufacturers of masks require different flow rates to produce set percentages. Therefore, care must be taken to read the manufacturer's instructions.

Implementation

Action	Rationale
Explain procedure to patient.	To help alleviate anxiety and gain co-operation.

Place patient in optimum position, usually upright.	To facilitate respiration.
Clearly display NO SMOKING sign.	To prevent fire/explosion. Oxygen supports combustion.
Correctly assemble equipment	To prevent leakage of oxygen flow.
Humidify oxygen, if required. N.B. Must be used with 40 per cent oxygen and above unless conditions contraindicate, e.g. pulmonary oedema.	To prevent drying out of air passages.
Set flow meter to prescribed rate.	To prevent over-/under-oxygenation.
Ensure mask/cannulae are correctly positioned and comfortable.	To ensure patient comfort and safety.

Evaluation

Potential problems of procedure	Appropriate nursing action
Deterioration in respiratory function.	Observe rate and depth of respirations and note any dyspnoea.
Changes in mental state, confusion or disturbed consciousness.	Check rate of flow and equipment.
Dry mouth.	Provide adequate hydration and/or oral hygiene.
Ulcerated nose or ears.	Relieve pressure of appliance. Alternative methods of administration may be required.
Atelectasis and lung infection.	Water within humidifiers should be sterile and changed daily.

N.B. The patient with chronic obstructive airway disease depends on low oxygen levels in the blood to breathe. Extreme caution should be used when administering oxygen to these patients.

Adaptations for home care

1. Advise the family and patient of the danger with smoking and open fires.
2. Instruct family and patient on the use of oxygen.
3. Check that local chemist is willing to deliver new cylinder when needed.

References and further reading

Bardsley, P. and Howard, P. (1986), 'Corpulmonale and home oxygen therapy', *The Practitioner*, vol. 230, pp. 565–71.

Collins, J. (1976), 'Blood gases, rational oxygen therapy: air flow limitations', *Physiotherapy*, vol. 62(2), pp. 49–50.

Leigh, J. (1980), 'Methods of oxygen therapy', in J. Gray, T. Nunn and J. Utting *General Anaesthesia*, 4th edn, vol. 1, Butterworth, London, pp. 531–49.

McMillan, E. (1984), 'Oxygen therapy', *Nursing*, 2nd series (the add-on journal of *Clinical Nursing*), vol. 2(28), pp. 822–5.

39   Insertion of a prescribed therapeutic pessary

Definition

To insert a therapeutic pessary into the vagina.

Assessment

Action	Rationale
Determine specific personal/cultural requests and ensure their fulfilment, e.g. female nurse.	To gain patient's co-operation and avoid incurring personal or cultural offence.
Determine presence of pad and/or discharge.	To assess the amount, colour and odour of vaginal discharge/blood to evaluate effectiveness of treatment.

Planning

Equipment

> Disposable gloves.
> Pessary and applicator when applicable.
> Lubricating jelly.

Action	Rationale
Explain reason and nature of procedure.	To minimise anxiety and to promote patient's co-operation.
Obtain verbal consent for procedure.	To ensure patient's full agreement to the procedure.

Implementation

Action	Rationale
Place patient in optimum position usually dorsal.	To facilitate procedure.
Teach procedure to patient.	To enable subsequent self-administration of pessary.
With a gloved hand, gently insert applicator/lubricated pessary into vagina.	To facilitate introduction of pessary.
Reposition patient.	To promote patient comfort.
Advise patient to rest and avoid bathing for 1–2 hours.	To ensure maximum retention of pessary.
Ensure applicator is used only for identified patient.	To prevent cross-infection.

Evaluation

Potential problems of procedure	Appropriate nursing action
Soiling of underclothing as pessary dissolves.	Advise patient to wear a pad.
Risk of cross-infection to sexual partner, risk of reinfection from sexual partner.	Advise partner to seek medical advice.

Adaptations for home care

The above principles should be followed. The patient should be taught to under-take procedure if at all possible.

References and further reading

Jamieson, E., McCall, J. and Blythe, R. (1988), *Guidelines for Clinical Nursing Practices*, Churchill Livingstone, Edinburgh, pp. 304–5.
Reynolds, M. (1984), *Gynaecological Nursing*, Blackwell Scientific Publications, Oxford, pp. 30–3.

40   Pre-operative care

Definition

The physical and psychological preparation of a patient prior to any type of surgical procedure. Research has shown that good pre-operative preparation facilitates recovery.

Assessment

Action	Rationale
Assess the patient's anxiety level.	To minimise patient's anxiety.
	To ensure patient's safety.
Assess the patient's knowledge and expectations of the surgical procedure.	To minimise patient's anxiety.
	To ensure patient's safety.
Check consent has been obtained and signed.	This is a legal requirement and a medical responsibility, but to prevent unnecessary delays to surgery, the nurse should check that it has been completed.
Assess the patient's skin condition.	To determine the type and frequency of pressure area care.

Planning

Equipment

    Accurate identification band.
    Theatre clothing.
    Denture container.

Adhesive tape.
Security envelope for jewellery, etc.

Implementation

Action	**Rationale**
Explain the pre-operative procedure.	To gain co-operation and facilitate recovery.
Ensure patient is given nothing by mouth for at least 4 hours prior to anaesthesia (except under medical instructions).	To reduce the risk of inhalation of stomach contents during intubation.
Ensure prolonged periods of fasting do not occur.	Long periods of fasting without intravenous therapy could predispose to dehydration.
Measure and record baseline observations of temperature, pulse, blood pressure, weight and urinalysis.	To detect and report any abnormalities. To enable the accurate calculation of doses of anaesthetic agents.
Check that the correct identification band is worn.	To ensure patient's safety.
Carry out any specific medical instructions, e.g. an enema prior to colonic surgery, shaving a specific area. This last is a controversial issue and the wealth of research available is divided in determining its overall value.	To ensure a safe surgical procedure.
If shaving is to be done, e.g. to increase a surgeon's visibility of an area, it should be done as near the time of surgery as possible, e.g. in theatre.	To promote patient comfort and well-being. To minimise the risk of abraided skin becoming colonised with micro-organisms.
Remove the patient's make-up, and nail varnish.	To enable observation and assessment of the peripheral circulation.

		Checked
1.	Identity band on patient	
2. a)	Consent form	
b)	Notes	
c)	X-rays/E.C.G. } Present	
d)	Prescription sheet	
e)	Cross-match form	
3. a)	Dentures/braces	
b)	Jewellery	
c)	Make-up } Removed	
d)	Nail varnish	
e)	Contact lenses	
4.	Last time patient ate or drank	
5.	Urine tested	
6.	Weight (in kg)	
7.	Shave	
8.	Emergency cases – relatives aware	

If any of the above are not applicable write N/A in appropriate column.

Full signature of trained nurse responsible for checking above.

. . . .

Figure 40.1 Nursing pre-operative check list.

Ensure the patient is as clean as possible.	To reduce the risk of infection.
Ensure the patient is wearing appropriate theatre clothing.	To maintain patient's safety.
	To reduce the risk of infection and allow access to the site of operation.
All jewellery and prostheses should be removed. Wedding ring/cultural equivalent to be taped.	To prevent burning from diathermy and prevent loss of items.
Document the presence of crowns or loose teeth.	To prevent inhalation or asphyxiation.
Encourage the patient to void urine prior to giving a pre-medication if prescribed.	To ensure comfort prior to sedation and prevent the risk of bladder perforation in abdominal operations.
Prior to the patient leaving the ward, a qualified nurse checks all the details with the operation forms, notes and X-rays.	To maintain patient's safety.
The use of an agreed checklist may be helpful (see Figure 40.1).	

Evaluation

Potential problems of procedure	Appropriate nursing action
Ingestion of food or fluid within 4 hours of proposed anaesthesia.	Report immediately to relevant medical staff, as this could result in delay of the surgical procedure.

Adaptation for home care

This procedure is not applicable in the community.

References and further reading

Alcock, P. (1986), 'Pre-operative information and visits promote recovery of patients', *NAT News*, vol. 23(7), pp. 17–18.

Boore, J. (1980), 'Pre-operative information and post-operative recovery', *NAT News*, vol. 17(1), pp. 16–22.

Dale, J. (1984), 'Sterile pursuit', *Nursing Mirror*, vol. 159(23), p. 14.

Dunkelman, S. (1979), 'Patient's knowledge of their condition and treatment: how it might be improved', *British Medical Journal*, vol. 279, pp. 311–14.

Hamilton-Smith, S. (1972), *Nil by Mouth*, Royal College of Nursing, London.

Hunt, M. (1987), 'The process of translating research findings into nursing practice', *Journal of Advanced Nursing*, vol. 12(1), pp. 101–10.

Petterson, E. (1986), 'A cut above the rest', *Nursing Times*, vol. 82(10), pp. 68–70.

Winfield, V. (1986), 'Too close a shave?', *Nursing Times*, vol. 82(10), pp. 64–8.

41   Post-operative care

Definition

The care given for the first few hours following a surgical procedure.

Aim

To maximise the patient's comfort and to avoid the potential complications following a surgical procedure.

Assessment

Action	Rationale
Determine the condition of the patient prior to leaving theatre/recovery room.	To ensure patient's safety and continuity of care.
Determine from medical staff any specific instructions regarding the patient.	To ensure patient's safety and continuity of care.

Planning

This may vary according to Health Authority policy, and the type of surgery performed.

Equipment

> Preparation of bed area.
> Guedal airway.
> Oxygen and humidifier.
> Oxygen mask.

Receiver.
Tissues.
Suction equipment.
Intravenous stand.
Observation charts.
Stand for drainage bags.
Specific equipment, e.g. chest clamps.

Implementation

Action	Rationale
Maintain a clear airway.	To reduce the risk of aspiration and asphyxiation.
Observe the patient's colour and respiratory effort.	Any change may denote poor respiratory function.
Administer oxygen if required.	To maximise oxygenation.
Perform oro-pharyngeal suction if required.	To remove excess secretions.
Check/monitor pulse rate.	To detect any rise of pulse and fall of blood pressure indicating shock or haemorrhage.
Check/monitor blood pressure.	To detect any rise of pulse and fall of blood pressure indicating shock or haemorrhage.
Check/monitor temperature.	To detect a rise or fall indicating a reaction to anaesthesia/surgery.
Observe any wound site/drainage.	To detect and monitor fluid loss from the site/drain.
Monitor intravenous and oral fluid intake.	To ensure that hydration and circulatory function are maintained.
Observe and record urinary output.	To monitor renal function and ability to void urine.
Monitor effectiveness of analgesia prescribed.	To maximise pain relief.

Reposition the patient as appropriate.	To reduce the risk of excess pressure on any point.
	To promote comfort, and facilitate recovery.
	N.B. Patients undergoing prolonged operative procedures are at risk of developing pressure sores.
Maintain all aspects of hygiene.	To maximise patient comfort.
Provide explanation and comfort.	To promote psychological well-being.

Evaluation

Potential problems of procedure	Appropriate nursing action
The patient's condition is considered to be unsatisfactory by the nurse collecting the patient from theatre/recovery room.	Refer to senior nursing staff/medical staff as appropriate.

Adaptations for home care

This procedure is not applicable in the community.

References and further reading

Boore, J. (1978), *Prescription for Recovery*, Royal College of Nursing, London.

Croushore, T. (1979), 'Post-operative assessment: the key to avoiding the most common nursing mistakes', *Nursing*, vol. 9(4), p. 46.

Hayward, J. (1973), *Information: A prescription against pain*, Royal College of Nursing, London.

Stephens, D. and Bowler, J. (1977), 'The nurse's role in immediate post-operative care', *British Medical Journal*, vol. 274, pp. 1199–202.

42   Pressure area care

Definition

The alleviation of any of the contributory factors of pressure sore formation.

Aim

To promote patient comfort and facilitate cost-effective care.

Assessment

Action	Rationale
Determine susceptible pressure points (see Figure 42.1).	These vary from patient to patient, depending on their position and bed surface.
Determine the texture and condition of patient's skin.	The patient's skin is a good indication to their general health.
Determine which of the following contributory factors are present.	To complete the appropriate score chart, e.g. Norton, Waterlow, Douglas (see Figures 42.2 to 42.4).

Contributory factors

Continuous pressure

Action	Rationale
Encourage mobility, change patient's position, 1 or 2 hours.	To prevent capillary obstruction depriving the tissues of oxygen and

(a) Supine

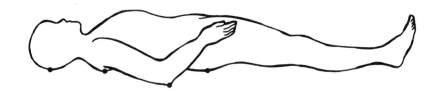

(b) Lateral

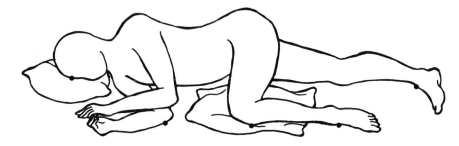

(c) Prone

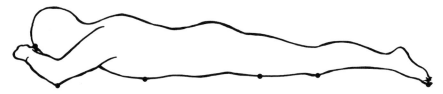

Figure 42.1 Susceptible pressure points.

Avoid constricting and rough bedclothes.

Use pressure-relieving devices, e.g. sheepskin, large cell ripple mattress/cushions, bed cradles and joint pads.

Shearing forces and friction

Action

Reposition patient in bed or chair, using pillows to support in a comfortable safe position.

N.B. Use of back rests can increase the risk of a patient sliding.

nutrients, causing a build up of metabolic waste. This will cause death to the surrounding tissues. Even short periods of continuous pressure can lead to eventual tissue damage.

Rationale

When the patient slides the skin can remain in contact with the supporting surface and the skeletal frame will move over it. Epidermal skin may be lost and superficial sores will develop.

A Physical condition		B Mental condition		C Activity		D Mobility		E Incontinent	
Good	4	Alert	4	Ambulant	4	Full	4	Not	4
Fair	3	Apathetic	3	Walk/help	3	Slightly limited	3	Occasionally	3
Poor	2	Confused	2	Chairbound	2	Very limited	2	Usually/ urine	2
Very bad	1	Stuporous	1	Bedfast	1	Immobile	1	Doubly	1

Total score of 14 and below = 'at risk'

Figure 42.2 The Norton score chart (reprinted by kind permission of Doreen Norton, the National Corporation for the Care of Old People and Churchill Livingstone UK Limited).

Immobility

Action

Change patient's position every 1 or 2 hours. Ensure that there are no creases or foreign objects in the area where the patient is lying.

Rationale

Some conditions cause the loss of spontaneous movement and pressure will occur.

Some patients have diminished sensation and will be unaware of damage to their skin.

Incontinence

Action

Change pads, clothes and bedlinen if wet or soiled. Wash area of skin carefully preferably using a non-irritant soap and pat dry. Apply a small amount of patient-designated barrier cream if indicated.

Rationale

Contact with damp items will increase risk of shearing.

Strong acids and alkalines found in the urine and faeces can damage the skin.

Frequent washing can deplete the skin's natural lubricants, causing it to become brittle and dry. Barrier creams can be occlusive if used in excess, preventing correct moisture and

Build/weight for height	*	Skin type / Visual risk areas	*	Sex / Age	*	Special risks	*
Average	0	Healthy	0	Male	1	Tissue malnutrition	*
Above average	1	Tissue paper	1	Female	2	e.g. Terminal cachexia	8
Obese	2	Dry	1	14–49	1	Cardiac failure	5
Below average	3	Oedematous	1	50–64	2	Peripheral vascular disease	5
		Clammy (temp ↑)	1	65–74	3	Anaemia	2
Continence	*	Discoloured	2	75–80	4	Smoking	1
Complete/catheterised	0	Broken/spot	3	81+	5	Neurological deficit	*
Occasion incont.	1	Mobility	*	Appetite	*	e.g. Diabetes, MS, CVA, motor/sensory, paraplegia	4–6
Cath/incontinent of faeces	2	Full	0	Average	0	Major surgery/trauma	*
Doubly incont.	3	Restless/fidgety	1	Poor	1	Orthopaedic – below waist, spinal	5
		Apathetic	2	N.G. tube/fluids only	2	On table > 2 hours	5
		Restricted	3	NBM/anorexic	3	Medication	*
		Inert/traction	4			Steroids, cytotoxics, high dose anti-inflammatory	4
		Chairbound	5				

Score:	10+ at risk	15+ high risk	20+ very high risk

1. Ring scores in table., add total
2. Several scores per category can be used

Figure 42.3 The Waterlow pressure sore prevention/treatment policy (reproduced by kind permission of J. Waterlow).

Nutritional state/Hb		Activity		Incontinence		Pain		Skin state		Mental state	
Well-balanced diet	4	Fully mobile	4	Continence	4	Pain-free	4	Intact	4	Alert	4
Inadequate diet	3	Walk with difficulty	3	Occasionally	3	Fear of pain	3	Dry/red/thin	3	Apathetic	3
Fluids only	2	Chairbound	2	Urine	2	Periodic	2	Superficial break	2	Stuperous	2
Peripheral/parental feeding	1	Bedfast	1	Doubly	1	Pain on movement	1	Full tissue thickness or cavity	1	Uncooperative	1
Low haemoglobin below 10	0					Continual discomfort	0			Comatose	0

1. Total score of 18 and below = 'at risk'
2. Special risk factors: deduct two for each factor
   e.g. steroid therapy
      diabetes
      cytotoxic therapy
      dyspnoea

Figure 42.4 The Douglas pressure sore risk calculator (reproduced by kind permission of Verna Pritchard).

oxygen exchange occurring within the skin. Multiple use of cream is a cross-infection risk.

Consider whether toilet training might be appropriate.

Re-establishment of a regular pattern of elimination should be the aim when caring for people with incontinence problems.

Diet

Action

Rationale

Encourage fluid and a diet rich in protein and vitamin C.

Record on the appropriate documents the patient's fluid and nutritional intake.

Poor nutrition increases the risk of pressure sore development and can delay wound healing. Supplementary nutrition may be required, e.g. enteral or parenteral feeding.

Body weight

Action

Rationale

Weigh patient and record on admission and at regular prescribed intervals.

Weight loss or gain may indicate a change in nutritional status. Thin patients have very little subcutaneous fat and will have higher pressure over body prominences. Obese patients may be less mobile and more difficult to lift and reposition.

Medical conditions which affect the efficiency of the circulation (e.g. diabetes, congestive cardiac failure)

Action

Rationale

Observe and record the patient's pulse (radial and pedal), blood pressure, peripheral skin colour and skin temperature as indicators of circulatory efficiency.

Any disruption of blood flow or volume will lower the skin's resistance to pressure and increase the patient's susceptibility to pressure sore formation.

Planning

Equipment

Select any pressure-relieving devices as appropriate.

Action	Rationale
Determine the most appropriate bed/chair that will promote patient independence and comfort and facilitate nursing care, e.g. flotation bed/cushion.	To relieve pressure. To prevent injury to nursing staff. To maximise patient participation.
Prepare appropriate equipment as determined by assessment.	To facilitate procedure and prevent unnecessary interruptions.

Implementation

Action	Rationale
Explain procedure to patient.	To gain consent and co-operation.
Maintain dignity and privacy of patient.	To prevent embarrassment.
Give appropriate care according to contributory factors.	To maximise patient comfort and reduce risk of pressure sore formation.
Maintain patient's hygiene.	To maximise patient comfort and reduce risk of pressure sore formation.
Ensure correct lifting and positioning of patient.	To maximise patient comfort and reduce risk of pressure sore formation.
Ensure correct use of pressure-relieving devices.	To maximise patient comfort and reduce risk of pressure sore formation.
Dispose of used equipment/linen according to Health Authority policy.	To prevent cross-infection and injury to staff.

Evaluation

Reassessment and evaluation of patients should be conducted each time the procedure is carried out. The use of a numerical score system can greatly assist in the evaluation process as it provides an easily interpreted baseline for reassessment.

Grade 1	Redness which blanches under light finger pressure, indicating that microcirculation is intact.
Grade 2	Redness remains, even when light finger pressure is applied. Blistering and the breakdown of superficial skin will follow.
Grade 3	Full thickness ulceration through to junction with subcutaneous tissue.
Grade 4	The sore extends into subcutaneous fat with lateral extension.
Grade 5	The sore extends through the deep fascia with destruction of muscle tissue. There may even be bony involvement.

Figure 42.5 Pressure sore assessment.

Potential problems of procedure

Development of a pressure sore.

N.B. This can range between discolouration of the skin to wounds of various depths (see Figure 42.5).

Inappropriate or faulty equipment.

Appropriate nursing action

Report and record appropriately. Determine underlying cause of pressure sore development and correct any preventable factors.

N.B. Pressure sores are always a reservoir of micro-organisms and care must be taken to prevent cross-infection (see Wound Care procedure in Chapter 56).

Ensure mechanical equipment is serviced at appropriate intervals. Check mattresses and laundered materal are firm and in good repair.

Adaptations for home care

1. The district nurse should explain to the patient and the carer the reasons for and the importance of pressure area care.
2. The district nurse should advise the carer regarding:
   (a) Lifting, moving and correct positioning of the patient.
   (b) Skin care.
   (c) Use of continence aids.
   (d) Nutrition appropriate to patient's condition.
3. The district nurse should advise the patient and carer of available pressure-relieving devices appropriate to their need.

References and further reading

Barratt, E. (1987), 'Supplement – pressure sores', *Nursing Times*, vol. 83(6), pp. 65–8.

David, J.A. (1982), 'Pressure sore treatment: a literature review', *International Journal of Nursing Studies*, vol. 19(4), pp. 183–9.

Gould, D., Leonard, M. and Baynes, V. (1984), 'Wound management', *Clinical Forum, Nursing Mirror*, vol. 159(16), pp. i–vi.

Hibbs, P. (1988), 'Action against pressure sores', *Nursing Times*, vol. 84(13), pp. 68–73.

Lowthian, P. (1985), 'Preventing pressure areas', *Nursing Mirror*, vol. 160(25), pp. 18–20.

Norton, D. (1975), *An Investigation of Geriatric Nursing Problems in Hospital*, Churchill Livingstone, Edinburgh.

Osborne, S. (1987), 'A quality circle investigation', *Nursing Times*, vol. 83(6), pp. 73–6.

Pritchard, V. (1986), 'Calculating the risk', *Nursing Times*, vol. 82(8), pp. 59–61.

Simpson, G. (1987), 'Assessment and choice', *Community Outlook*, vol. 83(27), pp. 16–18.

43 Psychological management of patients

Definition

Assisting the patient to maintain or obtain a state of mental well-being, concentrating on the needs of the individual and directed at the patient's uniqueness. Psychological needs include security; love, affection and companionship; recognition and praise; individuality; personal and sexual identity; respect; self-esteem; privacy and dignity; communication; knowledge and understanding.

Assessment

Action	Rationale
Determine whether specialist psychological support is needed.	Specialist counsellors may need to be contacted, e.g. prior to mutilating surgery.
Be aware of your own feelings and attitudes towards the patient and the treatment given.	Bias can affect judgement.

Planning

Action	Rationale
Develop awareness of the patient's history.	
Psychological support is based on knowledge of human needs. Prior knowledge of the patient will facilitate appropriate planning.	To ensure that needs are met wherever possible.

Implementation

Action	**Rationale**
Introduce yourself to the patient and explain your role within the health care team.	An introduction and explanation will help the patient to know what to expect from you, other staff and their stay in hospital.
Ensure the patient has the privacy and time they need.	To enable reflection and opportunity to communicate.
Show the patient that you accept and respect them as an individual.	To avoid stereotyping and labelling.
Determine the patient's perception of their problems and expectations regarding their treatment/admission to hospital.	To assess the patient's understanding and provide them with the opportunity to ask questions.
Encourage the patient to discuss their attitudes and feelings towards the proposed care.	The patient needs to identify and express their feelings. This gives the nurse the opportunity to provide reassurance and support and to demonstrate empathy.
Let the patient know that relevant information will be communicated to other members of the health care team, but that confidentiality will be respected.	Total confidentiality is not always possible; however, the patient has a right to know how the information is used.
Ensure the patient has the information needed to make choices, to question care, to assist with planning care and to embark upon treatment.	To facilitate partnership in care.
N.B. The patient may wish to include relatives and friends in this process.	
Be honest and consistent in all interactions with the patient.	To facilitate trust and confidence.
Give support and encouragement at all times.	To reduce anxiety and isolation.

Expect and allow the patient to be disappointed, sad or angry at times. Help them to express this appropriately and give support.

Inappropriately expressed emotion can delay the healing process.

Evaluation

Potential problems of procedure

Appropriate nursing action

Unresolved anxiety regarding:

- Altered body image/concept, e.g. hysterectomy, stoma.
- Discharge from hospital.
- The effects of treatment (see Discharge from Hospital procedure in Chapter 18).

Ensure other members of the health care team are aware of these problems. Refer to specialist counsellor/therapist and/or self-help group.

Difficulties related to honesty due to:

- Nurse's lack of knowledge.

- The patient who prefers not to be told the truth.

Seek advice from appropriate personnel.

Accept and respect the patient's wishes. Be aware that the situation may change.

- The situation where information is withheld.

Communicate with the individual(s) who wants the information withheld and find out why.

The non-participant patient, e.g. one who is unconscious.

Although unable to rationally participate in their care, the need for psychological management remains.

Adaptations for home care

This procedure may be utilised in the community as outlined above.

References and further reading

Grayshon, J. (1985), 'I want to go home', *Nursing Mirror*, vol. 160(13), pp. 26–7.
Orr, J. (1985), 'When the tables are turned', *Nursing Times*, vol. 81(21), pp. 24–6.

Schulz, J.M. and Dark, S.I. (1986), *Manual of Psychiatric Nursing Care Plans*, Little, Brown & Co., Boston.

Simsen, B.J. (1986), 'The spiritual dimension', *Nursing Times*, vol. 82(48), pp. 41–2.

Skevington, S. (1984), *Understanding Nurses: The Social Psychology of Nursing*, John Wiley, Chichester, pp. 74–6.

Summers, R. (1984), 'Should patients be told more?', *Nursing Mirror*, vol. 159(7), pp. 16–20.

44   Pulse (radial)

Definition

A measurement related to the expansion and contraction of the arteries as a result of blood being pumped from the left ventricle of the heart.

Aim

To detect any fluctuations/abnormalities in rhythm, volume and rate.

Assessment

Action	Rationale
Assess the condition of the patient.	To facilitate appropriate explanation of the procedure and to gain the patient's co-operation.
Ascertain the reason for and frequency of the recording.	To establish a baseline. To monitor the patient's condition without causing undue stress.

Planning

Equipment

> Watch with second hand.
> Appropriate charts.

Action	Rationale
Ensure the patient has been at rest prior to the procedure.	To ensure accurate recording.

Implementation

Action	Rationale
Place pads of first and second fingers over the radial artery.	To avoid the nurse palpating own pulse.
Gently compress the radial artery against the radius and count the number of beats for 1 min.	To palpate the blood flow through the artery.
Record on appropriate chart.	To ensure accurate monitoring.

Evaluation

Potential problems of procedure	Appropriate nursing action
Failure to detect radial pulse.	Attempt to detect pulse in an alternative site, e.g. carotid (see Cardio-pulmonary Resuscitation procedure in Chapter 11), brachial (see Recording of Blood Pressure procedure in Chapter 9), pedal (this may be routinely performed following some investigatory and surgical procedures).
	Report to medical staff.

Adaptations for home care

This procedure is conducted as outlined above.

Reference and further reading

Boylan, A. and Brown, P. (1985), 'The pulse and blood pressure', *Nursing Times*, vol. 81(7), pp. 26–9.

45   Rectal washout

Definition

The washing out of the rectum to remove faeces or prepare the lower bowel prior to investigation. Types of fluid that can be used:

Soap solution – 5 ml soft soap in 1 l water.
Hypertonic solutions – e.g. sodium phosphate.
Isotonic saline – two teaspoonfuls of salt to 1 litre of water.
Tap water.

The solution used must be prescribed by medical staff.

Assessment

Action	Rationale
Determine reason for procedure.	To ensure adequate explanation to patient.
Assess condition of patient.	To facilitate correct positioning of patient without causing further discomfort.
Assess whether it might be possible/ desirable to carry out the procedure in a separate room.	To preserve and maintain dignity and to reduce the risk of embarrassment to the patient and others.

Planning

Equipment

Trolley.
Funnel.

Rubber tubing.
Connector.
Rectal catheter.
Non-sterile disposable gloves.
Two plastic sheets and draw sheet.
Lubricating jelly.
Litre jug.
Large non-sterile jug containing warm (37–40°C) non-sterile washout solution.
Bucket.
Clamp, e.g. gate clip.
Non-sterile swabs.
Tissues.
Plastic apron.
Disposal bag.

Action	Rationale
Explain procedure to the patient.	To ensure patient's consent and co-operation.
Prepare the area around patient by placing a plastic sheet and draw sheet on bed and a plastic sheet on floor.	To protect bed and floor from contamination.
Position patient in left lateral position with knees well flexed, near the edge of the bed. Raise the foot of bed slightly if possible.	To facilitate procedure.
Ensure patient is covered by blanket.	To maintain comfort and dignity.

Implementation

Action	Rationale
Place bucket by bed.	To receive fluid.
Wash hands. Put on apron and gloves.	Reduce risk of cross-infection.
Attach rectal catheter to funnel and tubing using connector. Fill litre jug with fluid.	To enable measurement of fluid used.

Fill the tubing with washout fluid and clamp off when all air has been excluded.	Air entry into rectum may cause discomfort.
Lubricate rectal tube using swab.	To aid insertion of catheter and minimise discomfort.
Insert 10 cm of catheter into rectum.	To ensure adequate filling of rectum.
Fill the funnel with approximately 400 ml fluid.	More than 400 ml may cause damage to the bowel.
Hold funnel above rectum, release clamp and allow fluid to run in.	
Whilst there is still some fluid in the funnel, quickly invert it over the bucket and allow the fluid to run out.	To prevent air entering rectum.
Reclamp the tubing and fill the funnel with the same measure of fluid. Repeat procedure until fluid is returned clear.	To ensure bowel is clear.
Note how much fluid is introduced and returned.	The patient may absorb fluid, resulting in overload.
Ensure equipment is cleaned after use.	To prevent cross-infection.
Reposition patient, ensuring they are clean and dry.	To maintain comfort and hygiene.

Evaluation

Potential problems of procedure	**Appropriate nursing action**
Poor flow of fluid.	Move catheter around gently in case catheter end is pressed against bowel wall.
	Raise funnel slightly to increase gravity flow.
	Remove catheter and see if it is blocked.

Discomfort/cramps.	Check fluid temperature. Warm if necessary.
	Stop flow of fluid until cramps have stopped.
	Reassure patient to reduce anxiety.
Severe pain.	Stop procedure. Inform medical staff. Check pulse and blood pressure. Record amount of bleeding and observe stools.
Sudden onset of pallor, sweating, dizziness. Haemorrhage.	Stop procedure. Inform medical staff. Check pulse and blood pressure. Record amount of bleeding and observe stools.
Retention of fluid.	Inform medical staff.
	Record amount retained on nursing records.
A large amount of fluid is not returned after procedure.	Observe bowel actions to see if fluid is passed later and measure.
	Observe general condition of patient as patient may have absorbed fluid.
	Inform medical staff.

Adaptations for home care

This procedure is not applicable in the community.

References and further reading

Currie, J.E.J. (1979), 'Whole gut irrigation', *Nursing Times*, vol. 75, pp. 1570–1.
Hunt, T. (1974), 'Colonic irrigation', *Nursing Mirror*, vol. 139, pp. 76–7.
Lewis, A.E. (1965), 'Dangers inherent in soap enemas', *Pacific Medicine & Surgery*, vol. 73, pp. 131–3.

46   Recording of respirations

Definition

Counting the number of inspirations or expirations over a period of 1 min.

Aim

To monitor rate rhythm and depth of respirations.

Assessment

Action	Rationale
Assess if this observation is necessary.	To avoid the performance of an unnecessary procedure.

Planning

Equipment

One watch with second hand.
Appropriate chart.

Action	Rationale
Ensure the patient has been at rest prior to the procedure.	To ensure an accurate reading.
Wait until the patient is unaware of the observation.	To reduce the risk of patient altering their respiration.

Implementation

Action	Rationale
Count the respirations for 1 min by observing the rise or fall of the chest.	To facilitate an accurate procedure.
Record on appropriate chart.	

Evaluation

Potential problems of procedure	Appropriate nursing action
Imperceptible respirations.	Place the back of the hand near the patient's nose and mouth.
	Place the palm of the hand on the patient's chest.

Adaptations for home care

This procedure is conducted in the home as described above.

Reference and further reading

Boylan, A. and Brown, P. (1985), 'Respiration', *Nursing Times*, vol. 81(11), pp. 35–8.

47 Stoma care

Definition

The care of the peristomal skin and the safe, comfortable application of stoma appliances.

Definition of terms

Colostomy – artificial opening into the colon.
Excoriation – abrasions of the skin.
Ileal conduit – approximately 15 cm of ileum is isolated with its blood supply and the remaining small intestine is reconstructed to restore bowel continuity. One end of resected ileum is closed and the ureters implanted into it and the other end is brought through the abdominal wall where a stoma is formed.
Ileostomy – artificial opening made into the ileum.
Ischaemia – diminished blood supply to a part.
Urostomy – an opening into the urinary tract.

Assessment

Action	Rationale
Remove soiled appliance, noting amount and consistency of urine or stools.	To determine any abnormality.
Observe colour, condition and size of stoma.	To determine any ulceration, bleeding, prolapse or retraction.
Observe the condition of the peristomal skin.	To determine any redness, excoriation, allergic reaction or peristomal hernia.

Record observations in nursing records.	To ensure accurate monitoring of stoma.
Identify the type of stoma.	To ensure correct equipment is used.
	N.B. A colostomy in the descending colon usually requires a closed drainage system, as the stool is usually formed. All other types of stoma require a drainable appliance due to the frequency of action.

Planning

Action	**Rationale**
Assemble all equipment prior to removing appliance.	To prevent embarrassment and loss of dignity and to prevent urine or faeces having unnecessary contact with the skin.
Use a clear, drainable appliance for all types of stoma during the first four post-operative days.	To enable easy observation of the stoma and to allow emptying of the bag without removing it from the skin, thereby reducing the risk of skin damage.
Choose a mutually convenient time.	To avoid meal times, etc.

Equipment

This may be conveniently kept in a box at the bedside.

Appliance most suitable to the patient (drainable appliances require clips).
Template to accurately measure the size of the stoma.
Bowl of warm water.
Tissues.
Disposal bags.
Disposable gloves.

Implementation

Action	Rationale
Inform the patient of the procedure.	To obtain consent and co-operation.
Take into account the patient's preferences, e.g. bedside or bathroom.	This predisposes to individualised patient care and fosters the nurse/patient relationship.
Position the patient appropriately.	To ensure comfort and safety. To facilitate the procedure.
Wear disposable gloves.	To reduce the risk of cross-infection.
Empty the bag if drainable.	To prevent spillage of faeces/urine and enhance ease of removal and reduce the risk of cross-infection.
Measure contents.	To prevent spillage of faeces/urine and enhance ease of removal and reduce the risk of cross-infection.
Flush contents down toilet.	To prevent spillage of faeces/urine and enhance ease of removal and reduce the risk of cross-infection.
Remove soiled bag.	To prevent spillage of faeces/urine and enhance ease of removal and reduce the risk of cross-infection.
Assess contents (if non-drainable system).	To maintain accurate records.
Dispose into a plastic/paper bag.	To reduce the risk of spillage.
Or empty into the toilet before disposing of the bag into the plastic/paper bag.	To ensure safe elimination of waste without blocking the sewer system.
Place tissues under the stoma.	To prevent leakage of faeces/urine on to the skin.
Wash the stoma and surrounding skin with warm water and dry thoroughly.	To observe the integrity of the skin and to ensure a dry surface for the bag to adhere to.

Fit the skin protection or appliance snugly against the stoma. This may require the use of a pattern or template to achieve.

To ensure that no peristomal skin is exposed to urine or faeces, which could lead to skin damage.

Remove gloves.

Wash hands thoroughly.

To reduce the risk of cross-infection.

Evaluation

Potential problems of procedure	Appropriate nursing action
Allergic reaction.	Discontinue using the item that is causing the allergy. Wash and dry the skin thoroughly and apply calamine lotion and allow to dry. Apply skin protective wafer, i.e. stomahesive, and apply bag.
Excoriation of peristomal skin.	Identify cause of excoriation: • Check bag aperture correctly fits around stoma. • Check stoma has a spout and has not retracted. • Check if appropriate bag is being used and is correctly applied. Treat excoriation with calamine lotion and use a skin protective wafer.
Flatus.	Use a filter on the stoma bag. Give dietary advice.
Prolapse.	Fit a bag large enough to accommodate the stoma. Prolapses are usually reduceable but require corrective surgery. Inform medical staff.
Retraction of stoma.	Fit firm, rigid flange on to a one-piece bag to depress peristomal skin. Will require surgical refashioning and resiting. Inform medical staff.

Mechanical trauma to skin or stoma.	The bag should be removed gently and as infrequently as possible (a two-piece system allows the skin to be untouched for four to five days).

Avoid the use of a belt, which might cause friction. |
Bleeding.	A small amount of bleeding might occur when the stoma is wiped. This is normal. Bleeding from the lumen should be thoroughly investigated by the medical staff.
Ischaemia.	Observe stoma every 4 hours in immediate post-operative period. Check the bag is the correct size, so that it fits comfortably around the stoma.
Peristomal hernia.	This type of hernia rarely strangulates. A support corset can be supplied for the elderly patient unfit for surgery, otherwise surgical repair and resiting of the stoma is necessary.

Adaptations for home care

1. Store equipment in a safe, convenient place.
2. Prepare and protect working surfaces to prevent damage.
3. If disposal of used bags is a problem, arrangements should be made for collection according to Health Authority policy.
4. The patient/relative should be encouraged to undertake procedure at the earliest possible opportunity to promote independence.

References and further reading

Devlin, H.B., Plant, J.A. and Griffin, M. (1971), 'Aftermath of surgery for rectal cancer', *British Medical Journal*, vol. 3(5771), pp. 413–18.
Elcoat, C. (1986), *Stoma Care Nursing*, Bailliere Tindall, London.
MacDonald, L.D. (1982), *Cancer Patients and the Community – Outcomes of Care and Quality of Survival in Rectal Cancer*, DHSS Report.
Webb, P. (1985), 'Getting it right – patient teaching', *Nursing*, vol. 2(38), pp. 1125–7.

48   Principles of caring for the suicidal patient

Definition

Suicidal ideas are defined as thoughts of committing suicide or thoughts of ways to commit suicide. A suicide attempt is self-destructive behaviour that is potentially lethal. N.B. This procedure should be read in conjunction with the procedure for care of the depressed patient (see Chapter 17).

Assessment

The risk of suicide is increased when there is evidence of:

- A past attempt or when there are plans or ideas of suicide.
- Low self-esteem.
- No expression of thoughts or hope for the future.
- Perceived or actual loss, e.g. unemployment, change in body image.
- Lack of support by family or friends (particularly divorced, widowed or separated).
- Sudden change in mood or activity.

Planning

Action	Rationale
Assess the appropriate level of precautions necessary, using assessment data.	The physical safety of the patient is a priority.
Implement appropriate precautions immediately upon admission and daily thereafter.	Responsibility for the patient's safety begins on admission and their suicidal potential may vary.

Suggested levels of precaution are:

Level 1

The patient has one-to-one contact with an identified member of staff at all times, including visits to the bathroom and while sleeping.

The patient who is a high risk needs constant supervision and limitation of opportunities to harm themself.

Level 2

The patient has one-to-one contact with an identified member of staff at all times but may attend activities off the ward maintaining one-to-one contact.

The patient is at somewhat lower risk of suicide and movements are therefore less restricted.

If the patient leaves the ward, information and responsibility regarding the patient must be transferred.

Designating responsibility for observation of the patient to a specific person minimises the possibility that the patient will be inadequately supervised.

Level 3

The patient's whereabouts and activities on the ward should be known at all times. The patient must be accompanied by a staff member whilst off the ward.

The patient with a lower level of suicide risk still requires observation although one-to-one contact may not be necessary.

Be alert to sharp objects and other potentially dangerous items, e.g. glass containers or matches; these items should not be in the patient's possession. Watch for dangers in environment, e.g. electrical outlets, bed clothes, etc.

Determination to commit suicide may lead the patient to use even common objects in self-destructive ways. Many seemingly innocuous items can be used, some lethally. The patient may manipulate other patients or visitors to obtain dangerous items.

Avoid rooms at the end of a hallway or near the exit, elevator or stairwell.

The patient at risk needs to be closely observed to limit the opportunity for self-harm.

Implementation

Action

Maintain especially close supervision of the patient at times of decreased

Rationale

Risk of suicide increases when there is a decrease of observation by staff.

staff (nursing report at the change of shift, mealtimes, weekends and at night). Be aware of the patient during any disturbance or distraction and when patients are going to or from activities.

Encourage and support the patient to interact with other patients or to attend activities.	The patient's ability to interact with others is impaired.
Tell the patient that, while you are willing to discuss their feelings or other topics, you will not discuss prior suicide attempts. Discourage such conversations with other patients.	Reinforcement given to suicidal ideas must be minimised. However, the patient needs to identify and express the feelings underlying suicidal behaviour.
Do not belittle any prior suicide attempts.	Individuals who make suicidal gestures are gambling with death and need help.
Encourage the patient to express their feelings; remain non-judgemental.	Self-destructive behaviour can be the result of anger turned inward. Ventilation of feelings can help the patient to identify, work through and accept them even if they are painful or uncomfortable.
Do not joke, belittle or make insensitive remarks such as 'Everybody really wants to live'.	The patient's ability to understand humour is impaired. The patient's feelings are real and he may not want to live. Such remarks may alienate and contribute to the patient's lack of self-esteem.
Provide opportunities for the patient to succeed and give positive feedback even for very small accomplishments.	Positive feedback can enhance self-esteem. The patient's ability to concentrate, to complete small tasks and to interact with others may be impaired.
Help the patient identify positive aspects about themself, other people and their vocational life situation.	The patient's ability to recognise the positive can be impaired.

Evaluation

Evaluation of the patient should be ongoing and is of paramount importance in the early detection of a deterioration in emotional well-being.

Potential problems of procedure	Appropriate nursing action
Relatives' distress.	Support and provide ongoing information and reassurance.
The nurse's fear of the suicidal patient.	Provide support mechanism for staff, especially during periods of surveillance.

Adaptations for home care

This procedure relates to the care of the suicidal patient in a hospital setting.

References and further reading

Furness, J., Khan, M.C. and Pickens, P.T. (1985), *Unemployment and Parasuicide in Hartlepool Health Trends*, vol. 17, pp. 21–4.

Hawton, K. (1987), 'Assessment of suicide risk', *British Journal of Psychiatry*, vol. 150, pp. 145–53.

Schultz, J.M. and Dark, S. (1986), *Manual of Psychiatric Nursing Care Plans*, Little, Brown & Co., Boston.

Stuart, G.W. and Sundeen, S.J. (1983), *Principles and Practice of Psychiatric Nursing*, 2nd edn, C.V. Mosby, St. Louis, Miss.

49   Use of syringe pumps

Definition

The use of a specially calibrated syringe to administer a drug at a constant controlled rate.

Aims

1. To maintain constant blood levels of a drug.
2. To administer a drug in a small amount of fluid when using an intravenous infusion is contraindicated due to the risk of fluid overload.
3. To administer a drug, the side effects of which may be dangerous or unpleasant if given as a bolus injection.

Assessment

Action	Rationale
Check patient for known allergies.	To ensure patient safety.
Check cannula site and flush with saline if necessary.	To ensure patency of cannula and to prevent damage at the access site.

Planning

Equipment

Syringe pump, appropriately calibrated for specific requirements.
Syringe and needle of appropriate size, to be used in conjunction with the pump.
Extension line with Luer lock connections.
Dilution fluid for injection.

Syringe and needle (to draw up drug).
Alcohol-based swab.
Drug additive label.
Saline for injection, (for flushing cannula).
The prescribed drug.
The patient's prescription sheet.

Action	Rationale
Ensure adequate staff are available to check the drug safely.	To prevent misadministration of a drug and to adhere to Health Authority policy.
N.B. Two nurses, one accountable nurse and one other, are required to initiate and complete this procedure (see Oral Drug administration procedure, Chapter 36).	

Implementation

Action	Rationale
Check drug and dilutent (if required) against the patient's prescription sheet.	To ensure patient safety and to prevent misadministration of drug.
Maintaining asepsis, draw up the correct dosage using the small syringe and needle (use a dilutent if required).	To ensure accuracy and to prevent infection.
To set up a syringe pump:	
Draw up required amount of dilutent into main syringe.	To facilitate accurate administration of the drug.
Gently withdraw plunger of the main syringe.	To create sufficient air space to accommodate the drug.
Maintaining asepsis, remove needle and its protective cover from the syringe.	To allow drug to be injected into the barrel of the syringe.
N.B. Extreme caution should be taken to prevent injury to the nurse.	
Inject the drug via the needle port into the barrel of the syringe.	

Replace needle and its protective cover and invert the syringe to mix the contents (i.e. minimum of ten invertions are required).	To ensure a solution of even concentration.
Label the syringe.	To allow identification of the infusion for all personnel.
Remove the needle from the syringe and connect the extension line, keeping the 'patient end' sterile.	To facilitate connection of equipment to the patient.
Carefully purge the syringe and extension line with solution.	To ensure the line is free from air.
Check patient's name band against drug chart.	To ensure drug is given to the correct patient.
Fit syringe into pump.	To commence infusion at the prescribed rate.
Connect extension line to patient's access.	To commence infusion at the prescribed rate.
Set pump to required rate.	To commence infusion at the prescribed rate.
Switch on pump (two nurses are required).	To commence infusion at the prescribed rate.
Record on the appropriate documentation.	To ensure safe practice.

Evaluation

Regular review of the syringe pump during administration of drug is essential to determine potential problems at earliest opportunity (see Oral Drug Administration procedure, Chapter 36).

Potential problems of procedure	**Appropriate nursing action**
Inflammation of cannula site.	Stop the infusion and inform medical staff.

Cessation of infusion due to failure of pump (a warning signal may be given).

Check:

- The access site for swelling or inflammation.
- The pump for obvious causes of failure.
- The level of fluid in the syringe. Pump will stop when empty.
- The tubing for kinking.

Inform medical staff if solution is not readily found.

Potential restricted activity for the patient.

The patient should be encouraged as their condition allows to mobilise and be shown how to transport their pump appropriately.

Adaptations for home care

This procedure is not applicable in the community as it is related to intravenous drug administration.

References and further reading

Armstrong, E.P. *et al.* (1985), 'Clinical Comparison of three volumetric infusion pumps', NITA, vol. 8(4), pp. 305–8.

Coggin, S. (1987), 'Evaluating and selecting intravenous equipment', NITA, vol. 10(1), pp. 52–60.

Crow, S. (1987), 'Infection risk in intravenous therapy', NITA, vol. 10(2), pp. 101–5.

Engler, M.M. and Engler, M.B. (1986), 'Comparative evaluation of intravenous therapy regulating devices', *Heart and Lung*, vol. 15, pp. 262–7.

Jarrard, C. *et al.* (1987), 'The syringe infusion pump system – its affect on phlebitis rates', NITA, vol. 10(1), pp. 29–33.

Koszuta, L.E. (1984), 'Choosing the right infusion control device for your patient', *Nursing*, vol. 14(3), pp. 55–6.

Latham, J. (1987), 'Syringe drivers in pain control', *Professional Nurse*, vol. 2(7), pp. 207–9.

Ledger, T. (1986), 'Administering heparin with syringe pumps', *Professional Nurse*, vol. 1(7), pp. 176–7.

Moriaty-Sheehan, M. (1986), 'Clearing up infusion pump problems', *Registered Nurse*, vol. 49(7), pp. 40–1.

Rogers, B. (1986), 'Infusion pump programmes ensure safe intravenous usage', *Dimensions in Health Service*, vol. 63(1), p. 29.

50 Taking and recording of temperature

Definition

The measurement of human body heat.

Aim

To determine a baseline upon which to base subsequent observations as an indicator of physical health or potential threat to health.

Assessment

Action	Rationale
Assess condition and ability of the patient to establish method and site of taking temperature.	To establish method and site of taking temperature, thus ensuring safe practice.
	To establish the necessity and frequency of recording.
Consider normal range of temperature and normal circadian rhythm fluctuations.	The core body temperature in normal adults exhibits a low recording from 7.00 to 9.00 a.m. and a high recording from 4.00 to 6.00 p.m.
Assess patient activity and environment.	May affect accuracy of recording.

Action	Rationale
Ensure the patient has had no oral fluid, oral care or has smoked within the last half hour (oral route only).	These could alter the oral temperature.

Planning

Equipment

Appropriate glass thermometer or probe and electronic device.
Seventy per cent isopropyl alcohol swab or probe cover.
Box of tissues.
Disposal bag.
Lubricating jelly (for rectal thermometer only).
Watch.

Action	Rationale
Explain the procedure to patient.	To ensure co-operation and safety.
Ensure privacy.	Removal of clothing may be necessary to record the axillary or rectal temperature.
Select the correct thermometer according to site.	To maximise cleanliness.

Implementation

Action	Rationale
Clean the thermometer/probe with alcohol swab or encase probe in disposable cover.	Prevention of infection and cross-infection.
Ensure thermometer is ready for use.	To facilitate accurate recording.
Gain patient's co-operation.	To ensure patient's safety.
Place the thermometer/probe in correct position.	
Orally – under lateral frenulum (see Figure 50.1).	To maximise accuracy of recording.
Axilla – between two skin surfaces.	
Rectal – 2–3 cm anterially.	
Ensure thermometer/probe remains in position throughout the procedure.	To maximise accuracy of recordings.

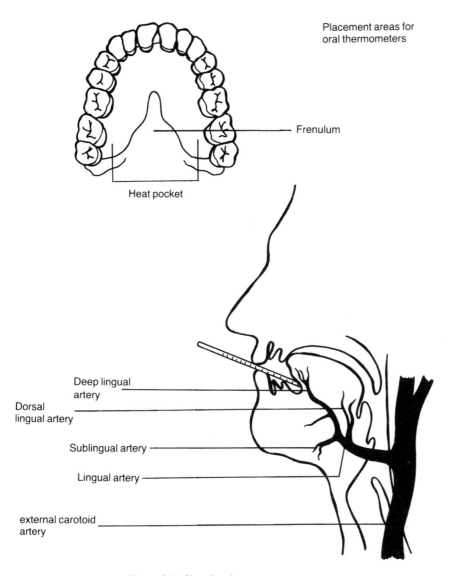

Placement areas for
oral thermometers

Frenulum

Heat pocket

Deep lingual
artery

Dorsal
lingual artery

Sublingual artery

Lingual artery

external carotoid
artery

Figure 50.1 Site of oral temperature measurement.

N.B. When the patient is restless, they should be supervised throughout the procedure.

To ensure patient's safety.

Ensure thermometer/probe remains in position for the correct length of time.

To maximise accuracy of recording.

N.B. Glass thermometers should remain in position for at least 8 min in every site.

Remove thermometer/probe and determine temperature.	
Clean thermometer/probe using alcohol-based swab.	To remove debris.
Ensure dry storage of thermometer.	To prevent multiplication of bacteria.
Ensure the patient is comfortable.	
Record/graph the temperature measurement.	To facilitate accurate monitoring of patient's condition.

Additional information for rectal temperature recording

Action	Rationale
Place patient in optimum position, usually left lateral.	To facilitate procedure
Select rectal thermometer/probe according to colour coding.	To ensure that the correct thermometer is used in the appropriate site.
Lubricate thermometer/probe cover.	For easy and comfortable insertion.
Hold thermometer in position throughout procedure.	To ensure patient's safety.

Evaluation

Potential problems of procedure	Appropriate nursing action
Breakage of glass thermometer.	Safe removal of glass into suitable container according to Health Authority policy.
Release of mercury during breakage.	Avoid handling mercury.
	Inform physics department.

Loss of thermometer into orifice.

Inform medical staff.

Faulty glass thermometers.

Glass thermometers can deteriorate with age. Check mercury line is unbroken. If mercury line is broken, dispose of according to Health Authority policy.

Adaptations for home care

If breakage occurs.

Safely remove glass into suitable container as per Health Authority policy.

Release of mercury during breakage.

Wearing disposable gloves, collect mercury into paper towel, fold towel carefully and dispose as per Health Authority policy.

References and further reading

Boylan, A. and Brown, P. (1985), 'Student observations – temperature, *Nursing Times*, vol. 18(16), pp. 36–42.

Campbell, K. (1983), 'Taking temperatures', *Nursing Times*, vol. 79(32), pp. 63–5.

Class, J. (1987), 'Oral temperature measurement', *Nursing Times*, vol. 83(1), pp. 36–9.

Ensign, J.D. (1972), 'Glass or electronic thermometers', Measurement Science Corporation, MED Issue 13.

Goodall, C. (1986), 'Heat trials', *Nursing Times*, vol. 82(8), pp. 46–7.

Hawkins, L. and Armstrong-Esher, C.A. (1978), 'Circadian rhythms and night shift working in nurses', *Nursing Times*, Occasional Paper, vol. 24(13), pp. 49–52.

Health & Safety Executive, (1975), 'Mercury, HM Factory Inspectorate Technical Data', HMSO, Note 21 (Rev).

McCarthy, J. (1983), 'Exposure to mercury vapour', *Occupational Health*, vol. 35, pp. 256–62.

Moorat, D. (1976), 'The cost of taking temperatures', *Nursing Times*, vol. 72(20), pp. 767–70.

Riley, J.A. *Research Report and Recommendations on Taking Temperatures in Hospital*, Sharoe Green Hospital, Preston, (unpublished).

Ross, D. (1984), 'Mercury poisoning', *Occupational Health*, vol. 36, pp. 215–18.

Samples, J. (1985), 'Circadian rhythms: basis for screening for fever', *Nursing Research*, vol. 34(6), pp. 337–79.

Saunders, F. (1985), *Temperature Taking: A study to compare mercury thermometer and electronic thermometer reading*, Hull University, (unpublished).

51 Tracheostomy care

Definition

A tracheostomy is a small surgical opening in the anterior wall of the trachea to facilitate ventilation and suction.

Aim

To provide and maintain a patent airway.

Changing the tube and inner tube of an established tracheostomy

Assessment

Action	Rationale
Assess the condition of the patient.	To facilitate appropriate explanation of the procedure and to gain the patient's co-operation.
Determine the type and size of the tube to be replaced.	To ensure correctly sized tube and inner tube are available.
Check availability of a pair of tracheal dilators.	A pair of tracheal dilators should always be kept by the bedside in case of displacement or inability to insert new tube.

Planning

Equipment

>   Sterile tracheostomy tube; introducer and tapes.
>   Sterile tracheal dilators (for emergency use).
>   Keyhole dressing.
>   Dressing pack including gallipot and gauze.
>   Cleansing agent – normal saline.
>   Barrier cream (patient-designated).
>   Sterile lubricant – normal saline or gel.
>   Sterile gloves.
>   Clean plastic apron.
>   Receiver for dirty tube.
>   Syringe, if using an inflatable cuff.
>   Disposal bag.

Action	Rationale
Explain the procedure and screen the bed area.	To gain co-operation and allay anxiety. To ensure privacy.
Position patient appropriately, usually upright, supported by pillows with neck extended.	To facilitate comfort and easy changing of the tube and to maintain a patent airway.

Implementation

Action	Rationale
Using an aseptic technique, prepare sterile field and arrange equipment (see Wound Care procedure in Chapter 56).	To reduce the risk of cross-infection.
Put on sterile gloves.	
Prepare the sterile tube by threading tapes and testing the cuff. The keyhole dressing may be placed around the tube at this stage or just prior to tying tapes.	To enable immediate insertion when required.
Lubricate the tube.	To facilitate insertion.
If a cuffed tube is in place, deflate prior to removal.	To facilitate removal.

Ask the patient to breathe out.	Conscious expiration will relax the patient and reduce the risk of coughing.
Remove soiled tube.	
Clean around the stoma, dry and apply barrier cream if required.	To remove exudate and micro-organisms – a moist skin encourages their growth.
Insert the sterile tube with an introducer using an up and over action.	Less trauma will occur if the tube is directed along the contour of the trachea.
Remove the introducer immediately.	To enable the patient to breathe.
Inflate cuff if required following manufacturer's/anaesthetist's instructions.	Over-inflation can cause damage to the trachea. Under-inflation will prevent an airtight seal.
Tie tapes securely.	To prevent tube from becoming displaced.
Place the inner tube in position.	The inner tube may be changed more frequently, thus reducing the risk of trauma to the stoma.
Ensure the patient is comfortable.	N.B. See procedure for Changing the Inner Tube in this chapter.
Clear away equipment.	
Clean soiled outer and inner tube and introducer under running cold water.	To remove debris from the tube.
If tube is very sticky it may need soaking in soda bicarbonate and water and cleaned with a small brush.	
Resterilise outer and inner tubes by returning to the central sterile supplies department.	To enable safe reuse.

Changing the inner tube

Equipment

Sterile inner tube of same size as tracheostomy tube.
Sterile gloves.
Receiver.

Action	Rationale
Wearing sterile gloves remove the inner tube and place in receiver.	To promote patency of tracheostomy.
Place sterile inner tube in position.	To promote patency of tracheostomy.
Clean dirty inner tube as previously described.	To enable safe reuse.

Evaluation

Potential problems of procedure	Appropriate nursing action
Blocked tube with dried secretions.	Change inner tube. Inform nurse in charge. More humidification may be necessary.
Displacement of tracheal tube.	Establish a patent airway.
	Inform nurse in charge.
	Determine reason for displacement.
Inability to insert clean tracheal tube.	Establish a patent airway using tracheal dilators. Seek help.

Additional problems of the new stoma (i.e. under seven days)

Tracheal bleeding whilst changing the tube.	Report to nurse in charge. Apply suction to remove blood from the trachea.
Increased risk of tracheal spasm.	It is advisable for two nurses to conduct this procedure.
	Inflate and secure new tube prior to cleansing stoma.
	A smaller sized spare tube and tracheal dilators should be kept by the patient's bedside.

Adaptations for home care

This procedure is conducted as outlined above. Tubes can be rendered safe for reuse by the *same patient* by boiling for 10 min. Many patients will learn to change and care for their tracheostomy tube themselves, once it has been taught by the nurse.

Tracheal suction

Definition

Removal of respiratory tract secretions via the tracheostomy for a patient who is unable to expectorate efficiently.

Assessment

Action	Rationale
Assess the patient's respiratory function.	To establish the need for suction and stability of patient's condition.
Assess the size of the tracheostomy tube and select the appropriate sized suction catheter.	If the catheter is too big, it will occlude the airway.
N.B. The diameter of the suction catheter should not exceed half the diameter of the tracheostomy.	

Planning

Equipment

> Suction apparatus, tubing and 'Y' connector.
> Sterile suction catheter.
> Sterile disposable gloves.
> Single use gallipot with sterile water for flushing.
> Tissues.
> Disposal bag.

Action	Rationale
Explain the procedure to the patient and ensure privacy.	To gain co-operation and allay anxiety.
Position patient appropriately.	To facilitate suction.

N.B. Normally upright for the
conscious patient. Laterally for
unconscious patient.

Suction pressure should not exceed   To reduce the risk of trauma to the
120 mm Hg for an adult. 60 mm Hg for   trachea.
a child.

Implementation

In the case of a permanent tracheostomy, every opportunity should be taken to
teach this procedure to patient and relatives.

Action	**Rationale**
Connect suction catheter to suction apparatus at adaptor end leaving catheter in packet.	To maintain sterility.
Wearing sterile gloves and with 'Y' connector open, pass suction catheter into trachea for approximately 3–7 in. (7.5–15 cm).	To ensure tracheal suction only.
N.B. In the absence of a 'Y' connector, the catheter may be kinked before insertion into the trachea.	
Cover 'Y' connector with gloved thumb, rotate and gently withdraw catheter.	To prevent trauma and facilitate the procedure.
Apply suction for a maximum of 15 seconds.	To facilitate respiration.
N.B. Suction should only be applied when withdrawing catheter.	To prevent trauma and facilitate insertion of suction catheter.
Flush catheter with water.	To clear suction apparatus.
Allow patient time to deep breathe.	To prevent hypoxia and unnecessary distress to the patient.
Repeat suction procedure as necessary.	To fully clear the airway.

Invert glove over catheter and dispose
into disposal bag.

To prevent cross-infection.

Evaluation

Potential problems of procedure

Appropriate nursing action

Excessive fresh blood on suction/
coughing.

Inform medical staff.

Apply oxygen via tracheal mask.

Apply gentle suction as necessary to
maintain airway.

Sudden deterioration in patient's
condition:

- Cyanosis.
- Air hunger.
- Restlessness.

Stop suction.

Inform medical staff.

Apply oxygen.

Check pulse and blood pressure.

Adaptations for home care

1. Ensure that a supply of sterile catheters remains in the home and the suction apparatus is in working order.
2. Prepare suitable working area.
3. Dispose of used catheter, gloves and tissues according to Health Authority policy.
4. Check that the carer remains able and willing to continue to undertake this procedure when necessary.

References and further reading

Allen, D. (1987), 'Making sense of tracheostomy', *Nursing Times*, vol. 83(45), pp. 36–8.

Allen, D. (1988), 'Making sense of suctioning', *Nursing Times*, vol. 84(10), pp. 46–7.

De Carle, B. (1985), 'Tracheostomy care', *Nursing Times*, Occasional Paper, vol. 81(6), pp. 50–4.

Harris, R. and Hyman, R. (1984), 'Clean versus sterile tracheostomy care and the level of pulmonary infection', *Nursing Research*, vol. 33(2), pp. 80–5.

Harris, R.B. (1984), 'National survey of aseptic tracheostomy care techniques in hospitals with head and neck and ENT departments', *Cancer Nursing*, vol. 7(1), pp. 23–32.

Jung, R.C. and Gottlieb, L.S. (1976), 'Comparison of tracheo-bronchial suction catheters in humans', *Chest*, vol. 69(2), pp. 179–81.

52   Traction

Definition

Exertion of a force onto a limb or part of the body. A counter force must be applied in the opposite direction to establish countertraction.

Indications for use

1. To overcome and minimise painful muscle spasm.
2. To ensure rest until healing has occurred, e.g. if a limb of part of the skeletal system is diseased.
3. To correct and maintain limb length where shortening may have occurred due to disease or trauma.
4. To maintain correct position/alignment.
5. As a pre-operative measure prior to internal fixation, e.g. fractured neck of femur.
6. To correct deformity.
7. To reduce dislocated joint.

Types of traction

Skin (see Figure 52.1)
Pelvic.
Skeletal (see Figure 52.2)
Skull.
Pulp.

Principles of traction

Action	Rationale
Elevate the foot of the bed (or head, if using halter traction).	To maintain counter traction.

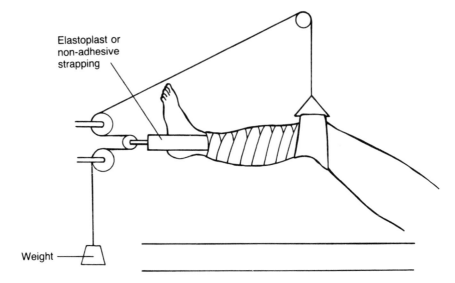

Elastoplast or
non-adhesive
strapping

Weight

Figure 52.1 Skin traction (Hamilton–Russell traction).

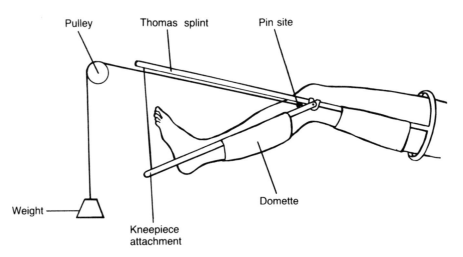

Pulley   Thomas splint   Pin site

Weight

Domette

Kneepiece
attachment

Figure 52.2 An example of skeletal traction.

Apply the weights and suspend over
an appropriate pulley.

Check correct amount of weights and   To aid healing.
that they are free swinging.

Check traction cord is tied securely and not frayed.	To maintain safety.
Check limb is in correct anatomical position.	To aid healing of fracture site.

Nursing problems associated with all types of traction

Potential problems of procedure	Appropriate nursing action
Traction sickness.	Report to medical staff. Reduce weights. Do not tilt bed.
Deep vein thrombosis.	Check for pressure around popliteal space and calves; observe for redness swelling and pain. Check pillows are in the correct position. Inform medical staff.
Drop foot.	Check for pressure around popliteal space.
Constipation.	High-fibre diet. Encourage fluids. Medical staff may allow the patient to use the commode if they are on pelvic traction.
Retention of urine.	Return bed to level position for toilet purposes. Fluid balance chart. Inform medical staff.

Skin traction

Two types – adhesive strapping and non-adhesive strapping.

Assessment

Action	Rationale
Determine the presence of any adverse skin conditions or allergies, e.g. psoriasis, varicose veins, etc.	To select strapping suitable for patient.
N.B. Adhesive strapping is not used for these patients.	

Planning

Equipment

Elastoplast traction set or non-adhesive strapping.
Two bandages.
Weights and weight carrier.
Pulley.
Balkan beam.
Strapping to secure bandages.
Tincture of benzoin compound.
Razor to shave the leg or depilatory cream.
One pillow.

Implementation

Action	Rationale
Explain the procedure to the patient.	To gain consent and co-operation.
Check patient is not allergic to elastoplast or tincture of benzoin compound.	To prevent allergic reaction.
Ensure privacy while carrying out procedure.	To maintain dignity.
Carefully handle affected leg.	To avoid pain and maintain patient comfort and prevent malalignment.
Shave affected leg (not required if using non-adhesive strapping).	To make removal easier and comfortable for patient.
Apply tincture of benzoin compound to medial and lateral aspects of the leg (not required if using non-adhesive strapping).	To protect the limb and increase adhesive quality.
Apply foam of elastoplast extension over the malleoli and bony prominences.	To avoid friction and pressure.
Apply elastoplast without folds or creases, one side of the leg at a time, from above malleoli to mid-thigh.	To facilitate application and to prevent discomfort and pressure.

Bandage the leg from above the ankle to thigh, using spiral or figure of eight technique (see Figure 52.1).	To secure elastoplast extensions.
Rest the leg on a firm pillow under the length of the leg.	To ensure even pressure and support.
Encourage exercises of foot and ankle.	To aid circulation to prevent deep vein thrombosis and a stiff ankle.

Evaluation

Nursing problems specific to skin traction

Potential problems of procedure	Appropriate nursing action
Allergy to elastoplast strapping.	Maintain traction and remove bandage daily and check limb for blisters or sores.
Patient complaining of parathesia or cold extremities.	Reapply bandage, ensure slings and pads are in the correct position. Inform medical staff.
Stiff ankle joint.	Active foot exercises every 2 hours.
Shearing of skin after removal of skin extensions.	Soak elastoplast with adhesive strapping remover and take off slowly.
Wrinkling or slippage of non-adhesive skin extensions.	Reapply as necessary, maintaining support and traction of the leg.

Skeletal traction

For a fracture of the shaft of the femur.

Assessment

Action	Rationale
Measure around the thigh, over the greater trochanter of the femur and beneath the ischial tuberosity and add 1 or 2 in (2.5–5 cm).	To ensure that the ring of the Thomas splint fits correctly.

Planning

Equipment

> Stirrup.
> Weights and pulleys.
> Steinmans Pin or Denham Pin.
> Cork or pin caps.
> Thomas splint.
> Roll of cotton wool or suitable padding.
> Domette slings to cover Thomas splint.
> Large safety pins.
> Traction cord.
> Knee flexion piece and screws.
> 'Sleek' strapping.

Implementation

Action	Rationale
Insertion of pin will take place in theatre in strict aseptic conditions under general anaesthesia.	To reduce risk of infection.
Apply weights and pulleys as for skin traction (see Figure 52.1).	
N.B. Sometimes leg is rested on pillows instead of a Thomas splint.	

Evaluation

Nursing problems specific to skeletal traction

Potential problems of procedure	Appropriate nursing action
Infection of pin sites.	Observe daily. Redress only if sore or discharge is present. Send swab for culture and sensitivity.
Ring of Thomas splint too tight.	Milk skin under splint hourly initially. Ensure it is clean and dry. Inform medical staff.

Pin slipping from one side to the other.	Inform medical staff and ensure stirrup screws are tight.
Danger of injury to patient and staff from sharp ends of the pin.	Cover ends with cork or metal caps.
Pressure sore on heel from slings.	Ensure heel is resting in the middle of a sling rather than over the edge.
	Relieve pressure every 2 hours.
	Observe for redness or discolouration.

Pelvic traction

Used for patients with low back pain.

Assessment

Action	Rationale
Explain procedure to patient.	To relieve anxiety and gain co-operation.
Measure patient around waist and hips.	To ensure correct size of belt.

Planning

Equipment

Belt lined with lint or cotton wool.
Weights and carrier.
Traction cord.
Pulleys.

Implementation

Action	Rationale
Explain procedure to patient.	To alleviate anxiety and gain co-operation.

Ensure patient is flat with two pillows under the head and one under each leg.	To ensure traction is maintained and aid patient comfort.
Apply belt lined with the lint or cotton wool.	To maintain patient comfort and reduce risk of pressure.
Attach traction cord weights and hang over pulley.	
Elevate foot of bed slightly.	To maintain countertraction.

Evaluation

Potential problems of procedure	Appropriate nursing action
Pressure sores due to pelvic belt.	Check skin under the belt for redness. Encourage patient to move around bed.
Paralytic ileus.	Inform medical staff. Restrict fluids and diet. Fluid balance chart.
Boredom.	Diversional therapy. Attach mirror to the head of the bed.

Adaptations for home care

This procedure is not relevant in the community.

References and further reading

Nicoll, K. (1964), *Understanding traction, Nursing Times* Publications, Macmillan, London.
Smith, C. (1984), 'Nursing the patient in traction', *Nursing Times*, vol. 80(16), pp. 36–9.

53 Removal of a vaginal gauze pack

Definition

The withdrawal of a gauze pack from the vaginal cavity. The gauze pack will have been inserted following vaginal surgery or as an emergency procedure for cervical haemorrhage. In both instances the pack is inserted to promote haemostasis. A gauze pack may also be inserted for therapeutic cleansing following the reduction of a procidentia.

Assessment

Action	Rationale
Determine specific personal or cultural requests and ensure their fulfilment as far as possible, e.g. request for female medical/nursing staff.	To gain patient's co-operation and to prevent offence.
Check loss per vagina through pack.	To assess and report the amount of vaginal bleeding.
	N.B. If loss is excessive, report to medical staff and leave pack *in situ*.

Planning

Equipment

Vaginal examination pack containing:
Sterile receiver.
Gallipot.
Sterile green sheets.
Cotton wool balls.

One pair sterile forceps.
Two sachets antiseptic solution, e.g. aqueous chlorhexadine.
A clean bowl containing warm water in which to warm sachets.
N.B. Dry sachets with a clean towel before use.
Sterile vulval pad.
One pack cotton wool balls.
Two pairs sterile gloves.
Alcohol hand rub for use between glove changes.

Action	Rationale
Explain reason and nature of procedure before and during implementation.	To minimise anxiety and to gain patient's co-operation.
Obtain verbal consent for procedure.	To ensure the patient's full agreement to the procedure.

Implementation

Action	Rationale
Ensure patient's dignity and privacy throughout procedure.	To minimise embarrassment.
Reassure and observe patient throughout procedure.	To maintain co-operation and position.
Place patient in optimum position, usually dorsal.	To facilitate procedure.
Cleanse and prepare trolley (see Wound Care procedure in Chapter 56).	To facilitate procedure and reduce the risk of infection.
Wearing sterile gloves, using gentle traction in an upward direction, remove vaginal pack and place into receiver.	Facilitates easier removal of pack.
Place receiver on bottom of trolley.	To prevent contamination of sterile field.
Discard first pair of gloves and cleanse hands.	To reduce risk of infection.

Wearing second pair of sterile gloves perform vulval toilet (see Female Catheterisation procedure in Chapter 12).	To keep vulval area as clean as possible and facilitate assessment of further blood loss.
Ensure patient is as comfortable as possible, remaining in the supine position for 1 hour following procedure.	To minimise risk of haemorrhage.
Clear away trolley and dispose of used equipment according to Health Authority policy.	To prevent cross-infection.
Wearing gloves, examine the pack for completeness with a trained member of staff. Record removal of pack in theatre notes and nursing records.	To maintain accuracy of records and comply with legal requirements.

Evaluation

Potential problems of procedure	Appropriate nursing action
Haemorrhage.	Initially check pad every 10 min and report excessive bleeding. Intravenous infusion is usually maintained until pack is removed and vaginal loss is minimal.
Retained portion of pack and potential subsequent infection.	All abnormalities should be reported to medical staff.

Adaptations for home care

This procedure is not applicable in the community.

References and further reading

Hector, W. (1980), *Modern Gynaecology with Obstetrics*, Heinemann, London, pp. 68–9.
Reynolds, M. (1984), *Gynaecological Nursing*, Blackwell Scientific Publications, Oxford, pp. 128–9.

54   Vacuum drainage

Changing a vacuum drain

Definition

Changing a container of a closed wound drainage system.

Assessment

Action	Rationale
Identify type of equipment in use.	To enable relevant equipment to be assembled.
	To ensure appropriate technique is used.

Planning

Equipment

Trolley.
Clean suction apparatus (see Naso-pharyngeal Suction procedure in Chapter 33).
Sterile vacuum drain.
Unsterile Spencer Wells forceps.
Disposable gloves (sterile).

Action	Rationale
Wash hands thoroughly using Ayliffe Taylor technique (see Wound Care procedure in Chapter 56).	To reduce the risk of cross-infection.

If non-disposable drainage container is to be used, apply suction until vacuum is achieved. Then clamp tubing.	To obtain and retain vacuum.

Implementation

Action	Rationale
Explain the procedure to the patient.	To reduce anxiety and gain consent and co-operation.
Clamp existing drainage tubing.	To prevent leakage.
Wearing gloves, remove old drainage container, maintaining vacuum by clamping at the container connection.	To protect staff. To maintain vacuum on the drainage site.
Connect new drainage container.	
Unclamp the system.	To maintain vacuum on the drainage site.
Remove old drainage bottle and measure drainage.	To ensure accurate record of drainage.
Remove gloves.	

Evaluation

Potential problems of procedure	Appropriate nursing action
Failure to achieve a vacuum.	Check position of drain. If holes in drainage tube are obvious, inform nursing/medical staff.
Risk of contamination of non-disposable drainage containers from ward suction apparatus.	Ensure suction apparatus is clean and dry. Use sterile tubing and connector.

Adaptations for home care

This procedure is not applicable to the community.

Removing a vacuum drain ━━━━━━━━━━━━━━━━━━

Definition

The removal of a closed drainage system, which actively encourages fluid to flow, under pressure, from within the body to a container outside.

Assessment

Action	Rationale
Determine reason for procedure.	To ensure appropriate technique is used.
Determine whether or not the patient requires analgesia.	To minimise discomfort to patient.
Ensure adequate space around the bed area.	To reduce the risk of airborne infections.
Close any windows.	To reduce the risk of airborne infections.
Remove any flowers.	To reduce the risk of airborne infections.

Planning

Equipment

Trolley.
Dressing pack.
Cleansing solution at room temperature.
Small-sized dressing.
Adhesive tape.
Disposal bag.
Alcohol hand rub.
Two pairs sterile plastic gloves.
Stitch cutter.

Action	Rationale
Select an appropriate environment.	

Wash hands thoroughly using the Ayliffe Taylor technique (see Wound Care procedure in Chapter 56).	To reduce the risk of cross-infection.
Clean the trolley according to Health Authority policy.	To reduce the risk of cross-infection.
Assemble the appropriate equipment on the bottom shelf of the trolley and attach disposal bag to bottom shelf of trolley.	To facilitate the dressing technique and reduce the risk of cross-infection.

Implementation

Action	**Rationale**
Explain the procedure to the patient.	To reduce anxiety and gain consent and co-operation.
Ensure the patient is in an appropriate position and as comfortable as possible.	To facilitate access to the drain.
Wash hands thoroughly using Ayliffe Taylor technique, or alcohol hand rub (see Wound Care procedure in Chapter 56).	To reduce the risk of cross-infection.
Open packs and prepare equipment on to the top of the trolley.	To allow easy access to the equipment required.
Wearing gloves, close the clamp on the drainage bottle.	To prevent backflow of waste material and to ensure safety for the nurse.
Release vacuum by removing tubing from the container.	
N.B. In some cases and on medical staff instructions, the drain remains vacuumed as it is removed.	
Cut the suture securing the drain.	To facilitate removal.
Gently withdraw the drain.	To maximise comfort.

Dispose of the drainage tube into the disposal bag, avoiding contamination from drainage.	To reduce the risk of cross-infection/contamination.
Ensure skin around the drain site is dry. Apply a small dressing.	To maximise patient comfort and reduce the risk of infection.
Wearing disposable gloves measure drainage and record.	To ensure accurate records and to maintain nurse safety.

Evaluation

Potential problems of procedure	**Appropriate nursing action**
Difficulty in removing drain.	Stop the procedure and inform nursing/medical staff.

Adaptations for home care

This procedure is not applicable to the community.

References and further reading

Cruse, P.J.E. and Foord, R. (1973), 'A five year prospective study of 23,649 surgical wounds', *Archives of Surgery*, vol. 107, pp. 206–10.
Lowbury, E.J.L., Ayliffe, G.A.J., Geddes, A.M. and Williams, J.D. (eds.) (1981), *Control of Hospital Infection: A Practical Handbook*, 2nd edn, Chapman & Hall, London.

55   Care of the potentially violent patient

Definition

Potential for violence includes the acting out of aggressive or hostile impulses in a way which may be violent or destructive.

Assessment

Action

Determine the patient who has the potential for violent behaviour.

The patient who has the potential for violent behaviour may exhibit some of the following characteristics:

- Body language, e.g. clenched fists, facial expressions, hedged posture.
- Verbal threats or abuse.
- Increased motor activity, e.g. pacing, agitation.
- Destruction of objects.
- Possession of a weapon.
- Self-destructive behaviour.
- Substance abuse or withdrawal.
- Suspicion of others.
- Inability to verbalise feelings.
- Vulnerable self-esteem.
- Provocative behaviour.
- Past history of violence.

Rationale

A period of tension is often felt prior to a violent outburst.

Accurate assessment, followed by appropriate intervention may help to prevent harm to patient or others.

Planning

Action	Rationale
Do not attempt to intervene if you are not appropriately skilled to deal with the situation.	Avoiding personal injury; getting help and protecting others may be the only thing to do.
	Exceeding abilities may put the nurse, patient and others at risk.
Never see a potentially violent patient alone.	
Determine that the patient has no weapons in his possession or within easy reach.	
If the patient has a weapon you may need to summon help from outside and pass the responsibility for decisions and actions over to them.	
Keep a comfortable distance, avoid intruding on personal space.	When an individual is in a highly aroused, anxious state, their body zone extends further than usual. Invasion into this space may be interpreted as threatening and provoking.
Maintain a clear exit.	
Be prepared to move quickly.	

Implementation

Staff should agree on reasonable limits for patient's behaviour. The patient should be informed of these boundaries and the reasons why they are necessary.	Clear limits let the patient know what is expected of them and increase feelings of security.
The consequences of exceeding these boundaries should also be stated and implemented if patient moves outside agreed limits.	Bargaining introduces doubt over the limits of behaviour.

Avoid challenges to patient's self-esteem.	The patient may feel helpless and inadequate. If the nurse communicates to the patient that they have worth and dignity, the patient will hopefully respond positively.
Avoid other patients being an audience to a situation. If other patients have become involved, encourage them to express their feelings after the situation is resolved.	Other patients may fear for their safety. Expression of their feelings will help them to feel secure.
Act quickly, using appropriately trained staff if it is necessary to restrain the patient. Make an initial assessment of the situation, then devise a plan for intervention before acting.	The physical safety of patients and staff is a priority. Firm limits increase feelings of security in all present. It can be reassuring to a violent patient that uncontrollable behaviour can be controlled and that harm can be prevented.
Determine adequate staff are available to ensure the safety of all present.	
Assign one person to restrain each limb. A fifth person, the nurse who has the best relationship with the patient, should direct the group and act as communicator.	Well-informed, confident staff will deal with the situation more effectively.
N.B. Remove own potentially dangerous items, e.g. jewellery, clothing, tie, watch, spectacles.	

Evaluation

Evaluation of the care given to a violent patient can be measured by changes in the patient's behaviour. If appropriate, the episode can be discussed with the patient, to facilitate learning and more appropriate expression of anger in the future.

There should always be a review by the staff of the episode. The aims of this will be:

- To encourage the expression of any residual anger or fear.
- To identify the precipitating factors to help prevent future episodes.
- To learn by experience the best ways to prevent and manage future behaviour.

Adaptations for home care

The above principles and practices may be applied to potentially dangerous situations within the home.

N.B. A district nurse should not visit alone if the patient or carer are known to be potentially violent. The nurse manager should be informed of the situation and the approximate time of the visit. The nurse should report to the manager following the visit.

References and further reading

Citty, D. (1985), A Validation of the Defining Characteristics of the Nursing Diagnosis 'Potential for Violence', Muns Nursing Clinics of North America, vol. 20, no. 4, pp. 711–22.

Schultz, J.M. and Dark, S. (1986), *Manual of Psychiatric Nursing Care Plans*, Little, Brown & Co., Boston.

Stuart, G.W. and Sundeen, S.J. (1983), *Principles and Practice of Psychiatric Nursing*, 2nd edn, C.V. Mosby, St Louis, Miss.

56 Wound care

Definition

Care given to a break in the body surface, caused by an accident or a surgical procedure.

Assessment

Action	Rationale
Determine the reason for the procedure.	To ensure the appropriate technique is used.
Ensure adequate space around the bed area.	To reduce the risk of airborne infection.
Close any windows.	To reduce the risk of airborne infection.
Remove any flowers.	To reduce the risk of airborne infection.
Assess wound size and site by observation of dressing in position (see Figure 56.1).	To ensure appropriate equipment is assembled.

Planning

Equipment

Trolley.
Dressing pack.
Cleansing solution (at room temperature).

Three sterile disposable gloves.
Alcohol hand rub.
Adhesive tape.
Appropriate sized dressing.
Disposal bag.
Any other specific equipment required, e.g. if patient known to have a bloodborne infection, sterile forceps may be used for this procedure.

Action	Rationale
Select an appropriate environment.	To reduce the risk of cross-infection.
Wash hands thoroughly using the Ayliffe Taylor technique (see Figure 56.2).	To reduce the risk of cross-infection.
Clean the trolley according to Health Authority policy.	To reduce the risk of cross-infection.
Assemble the appropriate equipment on the bottom shelf of the trolley and attach disposal bag to bottom shelf of the trolley.	To facilitate the dressing technique and reduce the risk of cross-infection.

Implementation

Action	Rationale
Explain the procedure to the patient.	To reduce anxiety and gain consent and co-operation.
Ensure the patient is in an appropriate position and as comfortable as possible.	To facilitate access to the wound site.
Wash hands thoroughly using Ayliffe Taylor technique or use alcohol hand rub.	To reduce the risk of cross-infection.
Open packs and prepare equipment on to the top of the trolley.	To allow easy access to dressing equipment.

Specific assessment for a patient with sutured incision/laceration

Name:

Type of suture:	interrupted	☐
	continuous	☐
	clips	☐
	tape	☐
	none	☐

Drains:

Type and number:	redivac	☐
	portex	☐
	corrugated	☐
	other	☐

Wound appearance – Location

Date										
	YES	NO	YES	NO	YES	NO	YES	NO	YES	NO
Clean and dry Localised tenderness Swelling of incision line Redness of incision line more than 1 cm Localised heat Purulent drainage Serosanguineous drainage	Signs of infection. Inform appropriate nursing/ medical staff.									

Figure 56.1 Suggested assessment sheet (based on J.Z. Cuzzell (1986), *American Journal of Nursing*, vol. 86 (6), p. 600).

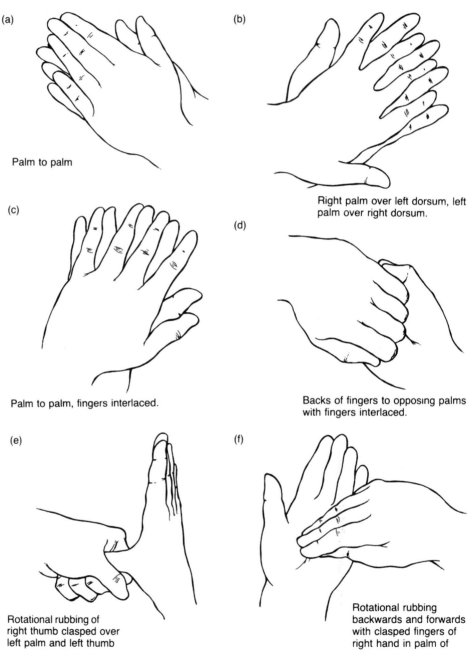

(a)

Palm to palm

(b)

Right palm over left dorsum, left palm over right dorsum.

(c)

(d)

Palm to palm, fingers interlaced.

Backs of fingers to opposing palms with fingers interlaced.

(e)

Rotational rubbing of right thumb clasped over left palm and left thumb over right palm.

(f)

Rotational rubbing backwards and forwards with clasped fingers of right hand in palm of left hand and vice-versa.

N.B. Number of strokes in each step is five. Hands and wrists rubbed till end of 30 second period.

Figure 56.2 The Ayliffe Taylor technique.

With a gloved hand, loosen, remove and discard old dressing, using an adapted Hampshire technique (see Figure 56.3).	To reduce the risk of contaminating hands.
Wearing sterile plastic gloves, remove debris from wound with gauze and cleansing solution.	To allow visual assessment of wound site.
N.B. cleansing solution may not always be necessary.	
Dry skin around wound with gauze.	To maintain patient comfort.
Apply an appropriate dressing.	To protect the wound and maintain an environment for healing.
Apply tape if necessary.	To secure dressing.
Reposition patient as appropriate.	To promote comfort.
Clear away used equipment and clean trolley according to Health Authority policy.	To reduce the risk of cross-infection.

Evaluation

Potential problems of procedure	Appropriate nursing action
Haematoma.	Monitor size and site and inform medical staff.
Localised tenderness.	Inform appropriate nursing/medical staff.
	Take swab or samples of discharge.
Swelling of incision line.	Inform appropriate nursing/medical staff. Take swab or samples of discharge.
Localised heat.	Inform appropriate nursing/medical staff. Take swab or samples of discharge.

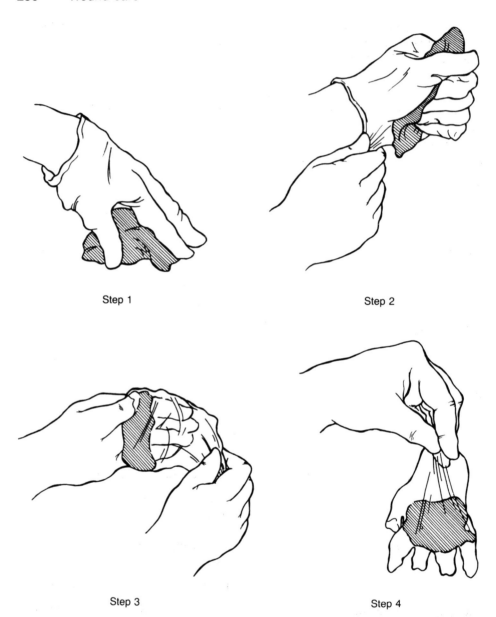

Step 1

Step 2

Step 3

Step 4

Figure 56.3 Adapted Hampshire technique.

Purulent drainage.	Inform appropriate nursing/medical staff. Take swab or samples of discharge.
Dehiscence of surgical incision.	Apply warm saline-soaked pad to wound.
	Immediately inform medical staff.

Adaptations for home care

1. Using the equipment available, appropriately adapt the principles and practices outlined above.
2. On completion of procedure:
   (a) Check that patient has an adequate supply of dressings/lotions, etc.
   (b) Advise patient/carer of any requirements, allowing time for prescription to be collected and supplies obtained from the chemist.

References and further reading

Ayliffe, C.A., Collins, B.J. and Taylor, L.J., (1982), *Hospital Acquired Infection, Principles and Practice*, Wright & Sons, Bristol.

Lock, P.M. (1979), 'The effects of temperature on mitotic activity at the edge of experimental wounds', *Symposium on Wound Healing*, Espoo, Finland, 1–3 November.

Taylor, L.J. (1978), 'An evaluation of handwashing techniques', *Nursing Times*, vol. 74(2), pp. 54–5, (3), pp. 108–10.

Thomlinson, D. (1987), 'To clean or not to clean?', *Nursing Times*, vol. 83(9), pp. 71–5.

Turner, T.D. (1982), 'Which dressing and why', *Nursing Times Wound Care Supplement*, No. 11, vol. 78(29), pp. 41–4.

57   Shortening a drainage tube

Definition

A tube which allows fluid to flow from within the body to outside, which may be removed by shortening in stages.

Assessment

Action	Rationale
Determine the reason for the procedure.	To ensure appropriate technique is used.
Assess requirements by observing existing drainage system.	To enable appropriate equipment to be assembled.

Planning

Equipment

Dressing trolley.
Cleansing solution (at room temperature).
Three sterile plastic gloves.
Alcohol hand rub.
Sterile safety pin (if necessary).
Sterile drainage bag.
Sterile scissors.
Sterile stitch cutter.
Non-sterile disposable receiver.
Disposal bag.

Action	Rationale
Select an appropriate environment.	To reduce the risk of cross-infection.

Wash hands thoroughly using the Ayliffe Taylor technique (see figure 56.2).	To reduce the risk of cross-infection.
Assemble the appropriate equipment on the bottom shelf of the trolley and attach disposal bag.	To facilitate the dressing technique and reduce the of risk of cross infection.

Implementation

Action	Rationale
Explain the procedure to the patient.	To reduce anxiety and gain consent and co-operation.
Ensure the patient is in an appropriate position and as comfortable as possible.	To facilitate access to the drain site.
Wash hands thoroughly using Ayliffe Taylor technique, or use alcohol hand rub.	To reduce the risk of cross-infection.
Open packs and prepare equipment on to the top of the trolley.	To allow easy access to the equipment.
Wearing one of the sterile gloves, remove any dressings, using the modified Hampshire technique (see Wound Care procedure in Chapter 56).	To reduce the risk of cross-infection.
Loosen and remove the drainage bag and place in the receiver.	To ensure the collection of all drainage for measurement.
Wearing sterile plastic gloves, remove any debris from drain site using gauze and cleansing solution.	To facilitate access to drain site.
Dry skin around drain site with gauze.	To maintain patient comfort.
Remove the suture securing the drain.	To facilitate procedure.

Withdraw the drain by the specified amount.	To ensure maximum effect from procedure.
Insert sterile safety pin into the drain close to the skin.	To ensure drain remains in correct position.
Cut off excess drain.	To promote patient comfort.
Apply sterile drainage bag.	To enable drainage to be collected and recorded.
Reposition patient as appropriate.	To promote comfort.
Clear away used equipment and clean trolley according to Health Authority policy.	To reduce the risk of cross-infection and prevent injury to staff.

Evaluation

Potential problems of procedure	**Appropriate nursing action**
Difficulty in removing drain.	Stop the procedure and inform nursing/medical staff.

Adaptations for home care

This procedure is not applicable in the community.

References and further reading

See Wound Care – Chapter 56.

Index